Creative Gro

with

Elderly Pe

DRAMA

DEDICATION

This manual is dedicated to Lorraine Fox and Roger Grainger, two exceptionally creative people I met at the start of my dramatherapy journey. They have remained constant sources of inspiration to mind, body and spirit as I continue to travel.

Creative Groupwork with Elderly People

DRAMA

Madeline Andersen-Warren

WINSLOW
Telford Road • Bicester
Oxon OX6 0TS • UK

First published in 1996 by
Winslow Press Limited, Telford Road, Bicester, Oxon OX6 0TS,
United Kingdom

002–3073/Printed in the United Kingdom

British Library Cataloguing in Publication Data

Andersen-Warren, Madeline
Creative groupwork with elderly people: drama
I. Title
792.0846

ISBN 0–86388–147–5

CONTENTS

ACKNOWLEDGEMENTS

There are a multitude of people I want to thank for their support, guidance and inspiration. First is my mother, who always encouraged my interest in drama. My teachers and guides include Sue Jennings, Gordon Wiseman, Ted Wharam, David Mann, Kath Yates, Chris Meredith, Augusto Boal and Marina Jenkyns. John Casson, Lesley McCallion, Jeannie Wright, Breege Laycock, Joan and Harold Mellor, Sue and Maggie Dorey, John Edmondson, Lambton Phillips and all of my fellow students on dramatherapy courses, Margaret Albutt and the staff of the Haven Nursing House, West Yorkshire have all offered friendship and different forms of support.

Thanks are due to all the people who have participated in my dramatherapy groups and training workshops and have so willingly ventured into the often unfamiliar worlds of drama and dramatherapy.

Finally a huge thank you to Hazel Krzywicki and Carol Reid who so patiently attended to the typing up of the manuscript.

FOREWORD

In this book Madeline Andersen-Warren shares with others her wide experience of working dramatically with elderly people. Her enthusiasm in helping them towards a fuller life is infectious. For some 'Age is Opportunity': relaxation, walks in the country and Saga Holidays. For others it means diminished faculties, impoverished role function and personal disengagement, which in turn may accelerate further decline. To use Madeline's own metaphor, she aims to bring the older person back from the 'wings' into re-engagement at 'centre stage'. To experience, and watch, in later years, the transition to failing autonomy can be emotionally traumatic to all concerned. It is just as painful a time as the emergent autonomy of adolescence and may deter those of a younger age from communicating with, and validating the experiences of, an older person.

Madeline's opening statements challenge readers to confront any negative attitudes they may hold about ageing. The detailed descriptions of how and why the creative activities can be used provide sufficient information to convince the reader of their wide application. The book is structured to take the reader through a carefully planned programme. Successful groupwork requires a professional approach, and that is how the reader is guided. The advice on preparation, including prior personal experience, leaves one in no doubt about the seriousness of the project to be undertaken and the care required to ensure physical and emotional security. Assessment, of the person, and of the issues involved, is an essential preliminary to groupwork, but one that is often passed over in an assumption that the leader knows what to do. The format given for assessing the client's physical disability is full and clear and includes some reference to mental disability. The importance of evaluation is noted.

Preconceptions that frail or hospitalized elderly persons, unlike the young, do not wish or need to engage in creative activities, are challenged and dispelled by Madeline's own belief that people can be creative regardless of age or disability. For her drama is essentially a pleasurable and creative experience which can transcend reality and the difficulties of the moment in a way that allows the rehearsal of new options during a temporary escape into an 'as if' world, with a later planned return to reality. Much of this dramatic world is verbal, but drama is also 'doing', a way of communicating through non-verbal meaning and experience.

Although written for the newcomer, there is much in this book to interest and assist people already working in the field. Not unreasonably, for relatively untrained persons, limits are suggested to the range of clients involved. Persons in the acute stage of a mental illness, those with severe dementia and those recently bereaved are excluded. While acute grief may best be avoided, some grief is likely to be shown in drama sessions relating to life events long past, and anyone undertaking this work should have a simple knowledge of the grieving process. In dementia the heights of imaginative creation may be precluded by cognitive and memory impairment, but there is still benefit and enjoyment to be found in 'doing' and in sharing the pleasures found in simple sensory experience.

It is rightly stated that Dramatherapy is adapted to many circumstances. Many of the 'warm up' and 'closure' techniques described are valid in their own right as a meaningful experience for the more mentally disabled. The complementary use, in dramatic form, of the patient's own life story through Reminiscence is noted and Validation Theory, an interesting related idea, is mentioned in the Bibliography.

A section is devoted to performance and covers a range of detail from seating arrangements that allow access to the toilets, through to script, props and costumes. Section two provides a progressive selection of drama activities including warm-ups, drama, text, puppets, masks, celebration and closures. The purpose of each activity is intended to be enjoyable, non threatening and potentially affirming for the participant. Section three, containing some useful addresses, concludes this valuable book.

Drama is a relative newcomer to the 'Therapies'. This book is a welcome stimulus to its use in a client group, that for years to come will present an ever increasing challenge.

DM & GE LANGLEY
February 1996

PREFACE

This is a manual for people who work with elderly clients in a range of settings: healthcare, residential homes, day centres, social clubs and drop-in centres. This may seem to be a wide area to attempt to cover. In fact, the scope of dramatherapy is even wider than this. Dramatherapy depends less on the physical accommodation in which it takes place than many therapeutic approaches, and one could go on listing social settings in which its approach would be uniquely valuable. This is because it creates its own setting: using the human imagination to construct a world of shared experience. The actual world is not ignored or blotted out — it is simply looked at in a different way. For drama-therapy sees it as the place you start off from rather than the thing you are stuck with.

The same is true with regard to being elderly: it is a fact, sometimes a stark one, but it is certainly not the only fact about being human, being a person. Elderly people, like young and middle-aged ones, have a part to play in the drama of life. What they say and do is as significant as what anyone else says or does, although they are not always encouraged to believe this by the way we are used to organizing things. Those who are not old yet can take a negative view of old people, one that concentrates on ideas of dependency and failing psychological and physical processes while paying lip-service to wisdom and experience. It is as if the older and more experienced players are given 'bit parts' to play in case they get in the way of the featured actors, or even upstage them.

Miss your cue more than a couple of times and you will find yourself confined to the wings … Even in the wings, however, the play goes on: here more intensely than ever, because of the limitations put on self-expression by nature and other people. In the wings (or the residential home, or the social club for the elderly), different ways may be found of playing one's own part. This manual, then, is for all the people who work in 'the wings' and want to venture into centre stage with their clients.

HOW TO USE THIS MANUAL

The creative structures described on the following pages are the result of collaborations between clients, staff and myself over a period of ten years. Many of them have been adapted in order to meet the needs of different groups, situations and settings. The activities outlined are not intended to be used as a 'pick and mix' assortment for random selection but as possible components for a safe and coherent group activity.

Like a thoughtfully and carefully prepared meal, the group structure could contain an appetizer or starter to whet the appetite, to stimulate the creative juices and to prepare for the main course, the body and substance of the group, followed by a closure that allows the components to settle and be digested, providing time for reflection and departure.

The success of a delicious meal depends on the careful selection and preparation of the ingredients, the blending of flavours, the dietary requirements of our guests and having all the necessary utensils for preparation and laying the table. We want to welcome our guests into an environment that does not give an indication of the hard work (pleasurable though this may be) that has gone into the cooking. The intentions behind this manual are rather like those of a cookery book. Recipes can be selected to form a meal but care must be taken to ensure that each course complements the others and that not too many flavours are produced. We need to serve enough food to ensure that people do not leave feeling hungry or unsatisfied, yet we do not want to put them off by offering to much. To start with, we need to serve food that people feel very familiar with before moving onto more unusual and adventurous cuisine. Very similar guidelines apply to creative groupwork.

Some participants, especially those with cognitive impairments caused by organic dysfunctions such as dementia, may not be able to engage fully with all of the activities described. They may sometimes become part of an audience, require more active staff support or intervention, or need some of the suggested structures to be simplified.

The first section of this manual contains an example of a general assessment form. It is not intended to diagnose or assess mental health problems. Procedures to establish cognitive function and to define any psychological dysfunction need to be carried out by trained personnel. Networking is always to be encouraged and the outcomes of any of the above tests should be available to people intending to facilitate groups.

Evaluation of the groupwork is also part of an on-going process of care and group leaders should formally communicate any results to others in the care team. Groups should not be viewed as an isolated activity, but as part of an overall system of care planning.

The manual is divided into three sections. Section 1 provides an overview of the possibilities of dramatic art with people of all ages and specifically with older people. It is intended to 'set the scene' for running creative groups and includes important aspects of the work, preparing yourself, others and the environment, and resources. It contains information on assessment, recording and evaluation and how to structure the groups.

Section 2 is intended to be read in conjunction with Section 1. It contains suggestions for group activities with this particular client group. Although this, the major section of the manual, is devoted to practical ideas, it is not the intention of the author that these should be implemented without considering all the preparation advice contained above and in Section 1.

Section 3 contains useful addresses, information on organizations and suggestions for further reading.

Author's notes

I am grateful to Dorothy and Gordon Langley for pointing out that, whilst informed consent is a very important issue with those who have the capacity to consent, there are large numbers of confused elderly people who do not have the ability to understand the nature and major risks of their treatment. Case law as it now stands is that doctors can act in the 'best interests' of an incapacitated person who does not resist.

If there is any doubt about a client's ability to give consent, advice should be sought from an appropriate agency. Organizations that provide advocacy services for older people will often be able to provide up-to-date information.

Madeline Andersen-Warren is at present a clinical nurse specialist/dramatherapist employed in a Northern NHS Trust. She initially trained as a stage manager and worked in repertory theatres before qualifying as a mental health nurse. Post-registration training included a six-month course on nursing the elderly client. Throughout this time she retained her strong interest in the theatre and later obtained a degree in Theatre Studies and qualified as a dramatherapist, trainer and supervisor.

She has pioneered therapeutic theatre forms of dramatherapy with clients receiving long-term care and also successfully introduced dramatherapy within a wide range of settings. She is a visiting lecturer at several universities and colleges and co-ordinator of Dramatherapy North West, a local network of the British Association for Dramatherapists.

The research she is now engaged in, for a higher degree, is based on her experience in clinical practice.

SECTION 1

INTRODUCTION

THE PURPOSE OF THIS MANUAL

This is mainly a practical manual, a sourcebook of material for those without specialist knowledge of drama or creative methods of working. It is not intended as a substitute for training. It is generally unwise to lead any creative groupwork without any practical experience of the media. There are a multitude of one- and two-day workshops in Britain (a list of addresses can be found at the back of this manual). It would be very helpful to have attended, at the very least, a two-day course on leadership of creative groups. The workshop does not need to be specifically about working with elderly people. It is important to become involved in a form of creative drama to experience the atmosphere of becoming engaged in the process, and to discover or rediscover one's own creative impulses before starting to work with others. If this is not really possible, gather together a group of willing colleagues or friends and experiment with some of the exercises in this manual.

A golden rule is never to run a creative group without some previous practical experience. After all, we would not want to set ourselves up as, for example, a sports coach without prior involvement in the sport. It is not enough just to know the rules of the game, we need to have the experience of 'being in the field' as well, in order to be able to communicate effectively.

The major part of the manual is concerned with suggestions for dramatic activities with older people. These activities include storymaking, working with texts, puppets and masks, and improvisation. A selection of group warm-ups and closures are provided. Each of the outlines begins with the purpose ('Focus') of the activity. Most of them are devised for running groups with people with a range of physical and mental capabilities, but it is important that they be seen as suggestions for activities and adapted for each particular group of people as necessary.

Before planning the groups, the leaders need to be very aware of physical and mental difficulties associated with old age that may present problems in regard to their relationships with other people. Someone who has difficulty walking will feel out of place, and probably be treated as such, in a group of ramblers. To this extent, the circumstances in which the group takes place are very important indeed and group leaders need to be realistic in their expectations about what is likely to prove an obstacle to the therapeutic value of the group. This does not mean that every member of the group has to have the same degree of disability, or any disability at all, for that matter. It does mean, however, that disabilities, handicaps and emotional or cognitive problems must always be taken into account, and never simply ignored. They concern the nature of the group itself, which is intimately connected with the circumstances of membership, setting, time of meeting and official or unofficial purpose. At this level the group *is* its members, even before it sees itself as a group or has a conscious identity as such. This is the raw material and any dramatic process, however simple, must start from this point. Five people in armchairs and one in a wheelchair will use this precise difference instead of ignoring it. It will both inform and enhance the drama, communication and understanding. But the group leaders must be aware of these points of similarities and differences between group members before starting to plan the drama, so that a shared starting-point can be identified.

Before including anyone in a group activity, the group leaders must be aware of the client's emotional and physical capabilities. They should liaise with other staff, and read carefully case-notes, care programmes and any other records. They must be absolutely sure that they know signs and symptoms associated with physical or emotional distress.

The drama

1. Allow people to participate at their own level. It is dangerous to force people to extend their physical or emotional capabilities.

2. The exercises suggested within these pages are designed to enhance well-being through the medium of creativity. They are not intended to be psychotherapy, which requires the skills of people specifically trained in that field.

3. The dramatic activities outlined have all been tried and tested. They focus on what we can create together as a group, to celebrate our strengths, our communications and our differences. They are intended to be life enhancing and must be experienced within a safe group atmosphere.

4. *Be careful* not to view the drama as a collection of techniques or games. The groups must be run as a planned activity with clear aims and objectives.

5. Always be aware of the potential power of the creative process. Sometimes uncomfortable memories or feelings

can be stirred. Ensure that participants have an opportunity to discuss these and that people do not leave the group in a distressed state; and make sure that they have appropriate support outside the group.

The organization

1. The group should not be an isolated activity but a planned component of a plan of care.
2. Ensure that you are not interfering with any other care or support that clients are receiving.
3. Ensure that all relevant staff, that is managers and other carers, know that the group is being planned.
4. Do not be tempted to give advice about any medical, legal or social matters. Refer such questions to those qualified to deal with them.
5. Be fully conversant with local and national health and safety regulations and any policies relating to creative therapies and record keeping.

The group leaders

1. Training is essential before starting creative groupwork.
2. Supervision by a trained supervisor who is conversant with and experienced in creative therapies is an essential component of good practice.
3. Careful assessment and evaluation procedures are essential.
4. Only include clients who have given informed consent.
5. Be aware of the way in which your own attitudes to old age can influence your relationship with group members.
6. Never try out activities with a client group. Experiment with other staff members, friends and so on.
7. Ensure that the aims of the group leaders are never in conflict with the aims of the clients.

Specific contraindications

Do not include people with the following conditions: acute mental health disorders; the later stages of any dementia; any physical disorders in which activity is contraindicated.
Do not include those who have suffered recent losses. **Above all the group must be physically and emotionally safe for all involved.**

THE POSSIBILITIES OF DRAMA WITH ALL AGE GROUPS

Drama depends on imaginative involvement. Dramatherapy, therefore, is a kind of therapy which involves imagination, and the kind of understanding about ourselves and other people that drama gives us. You could say that this is 'a kind of forgetting in order to remember', or 'losing yourself in order to discover yourself again'. We lose ourselves in a situation involving other people, in which we can temporarily forget our own anxieties and concentrate on someone else, so that we can rediscover ourselves as unique individuals, with our own destinies and our own personal contributions to life. Or we can use our memories of the past and ideas about the future to imagine ourselves as we were or might be at other times in our lives and other situations than the one in which we now find ourselves.

Our own situations, the things that happen to us, have the power to contain us, to make us feel trapped in what is happening now. Drama is different. It may involve us, but it cannot restrict our personal freedom. We are moved by what the characters involved are going through, but we do not have to go through it ourselves — except in our imaginations, as we identify our own feelings with theirs. The drama ended, we are returned to our own ordinary state of mind, to find it changed by the experience. Somehow, in the company of the people in the play, we have passed through the valley and emerged into the daylight. It was not a real valley, only an imaginary one; but the feelings it gave us were real enough, and we are relieved they are past.

This, then, is the fundamental principle upon which dramatherapy is based. It need not involve using actual drama, in the sense of plays that are ready-made for use. Whenever we find ourselves trying the world out for size, by using one particular set of circumstances *as if* they were another, we are involved in a kind of drama which, once it is applied to the lives of the people taking part, may allow feelings to be shared and insights explored. This is why dramatherapy does not always have to be approached in the same way, involving the same kinds of people. If we can use our imagination at all and can 'see this as if it were this', we can explore our own experiences in a way that we can cope with. The degree of psychological stress will always depend on how closely we have identified with the kind of experience that we are imagining. This is something we find ourselves able to control, however; it involves learning to 'temper the wind to the shorn lamb' in the light of clients' vulnerability to the power of suggestion.

Dramatherapists develop the flexibility to work with groups or individuals, same-sex or mixed gender groups, with people of any age able to imagine. More important still, they learn to use the differences between group members to the group's actual advantage, helping people to share across the barriers of age, sex, educational attainment — even medication sometimes! Within psychiatric settings, dramatherapy groups contain people who look at life in dramatically different ways, yet find a meeting ground in symbols that have been painstakingly negotiated among them; for each group, with the help and guidance of the therapist, discovers the kind of human material to work on which means something to everybody present. The fact that it will inevitably mean something different to each person only adds to the richness of the experience of sharing, for the group will create its own drama by taking into account everything that contributes to its own unique identity. Where diagnosis always divides — as it is designed to do — dramatherapy have a way of uniting.

Drama and dramatherapy both depend on the communication of experience. This is experience of all kinds, not only inform ation about specific events involving personal trauma. Crises leading to some kind of breakdown take place against a background of things that are ordinary and recognizable. It is the existence of a shared experience of ordinary things that gives rise to effective dramatherapy; and despite a tendency to forget what has only happened recently, elderly people have shared more of life with others than young people have, simply because they had had more of it to share.

DRAMA AS A 'THING DONE'

The original meaning of drama is 'doing', and this remains its basic meaning. Drama is communicated by means of actions that express meaning, artistically presented for the greatest impact and clarity. In fact dramatherapy involves several different kinds of art, which are designed to appeal to particular senses: speech and music, reaching us through our ears; painting, sculpture, light, movement and gesture, which we can appreciate visually; ceramics and fabrics that we touch as well as look at. Sometimes food may be prepared in ways that make eating and drinking a kind of artistic experience. Each of these 'sensory media' can be a way of enjoying what is involved in being a living person. They all bring us back to basics, giving us a kind of natural, immediate, sense of enjoyment of being alive. They can thus be sources of dramatherapy — the basic therapy of doing things that communicate living experience.

In other words, artistic creativity is a way in which we express and share our world, not by describing it but by actually *living* it; living it in a particular way that allows it to speak through our senses to us. Our works of art reflect us without imposing our experience on others. No matter how powerfully my music, sculpture or poem 'speaks', it cannot force anyone to agree or even listen. *We take from the experience what we ourselves want and give to it what we are willing to share.* All this, of course, refers to the way in which a kind of artistic experience provides the main medium for a dramatherapy session or course of sessions. We often make use of art in a secondary or supporting role to build atmosphere or to provide contrast or give depth to the main medium we are working with; or we build up our artistic 'world' out of material of several kinds, so that colour, sound, movement and textures all contribute to our ability to express ourselves through our own — and other people's — senses. Art, then, may be either foreground or background, or both.

Not everybody thinks of themselves as an artist, however. The great majority of us would be quite terrified by the idea! Elderly people are usually eager to say that they are 'past all that sort of thing'. They no longer have the physical dexterity or the ability to concentrate that they once possessed. And anyway, most people are not artists, and never were. It really is not fair to put elderly people into situations in which they will feel embarrassed by their lack of skill. Art should be left to the artists, whether they are painters, musicians or actors. Besides, a lot of people can remember having to take part in drama at school, and feeling very awkward and self-conscious about it, too!

Dramatherapists always have a lot of sympathy with people who feel like this. They do their best to explain that dramatherapy does not mean having to act in plays, and certainly no-one should be made to feel foolish or inadequate by taking part. Dramatherapy is made for the client, not the client for dramatherapy. What matters is joining in and having a go, seeing what it is like; dramatherapy involves exploring things and has to do with discovery and rediscovery. By beating out rhythmic patterns on pieces of bamboo we *become* musicians, and we emerge as new-born artists as we discover the joys of finger-painting. The place for artistic expertise is in setting the scene for the client's imagination to bring to life. Music, movement, lighting effects and evocative sound can all have their part to play in this.

As a matter of fact, for those taking part in the action, technical skill can sometimes actually get in the way, because it can introduce an element of competition into what is essentially a corporate experience. It is important that everyone travels this route together. In this way, dramatherapy is in itself a shared act, bearing witness to and embodying a shared imaginative experience.

DRAMATHERAPY WITH ELDERLY CLIENTS

Dramatherapy does not have to be specially adapted for different kinds of people. Each group will create its own kind of imaginative drama out of its own particular situation and circumstances. Dramatherapy with elderly people means what it says: this is dramatherapy as elderly people may produce it. The same would be true of 'dramatherapy with children' or 'dramatherapy with teenagers'. We always have to take people's capabilities, physical and mental, into consideration when planning groups, but this does not mean that the processes involved in the therapy are different. There is no standard 'original' kind of dramatherapy designed for people who have no special characteristics, and dramatherapy always meets its clients where they are and adapts itself to them. However, in this manual, we are looking at a specific model of dramatherapy. Jennings (1990, pages 27–46), defines four of these models:

1. ***The creative expressive model***, which focuses on the imaginative impulses and people's latent creativity.
2. ***The tasks and skills model***, which seeks to expand the behavioural repertoire.
3. ***The psychotherapeutic methodology***, working through psychological insights to produce change in individuals and groups.
4. ***The integrated model***, an advanced approach which combines models 1, 2 and 3 but works towards a deep level of psychological awareness through dramatic art.

This manual is concerned mainly with model 1, the creative expressive model, which can allow the expression of feeling through the creative medium. This way of working may include performance. The advantages and disadvantages of performance are discussed on pages 51–2.

The suggestions for activities contained in the following pages are intended for those who have not trained as dramatherapists. As with any other group of people, we should always be aware that the presence of distress of a recognizably clinical kind (that is, when distress is prolonged and intractable) may require specialized intervention.

Aims and objectives

'Aims' indicate the direction in which we want to move, and 'objectives' the specific standard to be achieved in that direction.

Physical aims and objectives

1. To enlarge and develop physical awareness and capability.
2. To reincorporate parts of the organism which, having been deprived of their operational function, have also lost their ability to transmit symbolic messages. (For example, patients who had lost the use of one hand as a result of a stroke would not on any account let themselves touch the affected limb. When, however, they were encouraged to make the imaginative leap involved in their hand 'becoming a beautiful butterfly', the paralysed hand was quite easily seen as a branch for the butterfly to alight on.)
3. To extend the scope of movement: drama changes the way we see ourselves; with new kinds of roles we find ourselves moving in ways that are new. (For example, a woman with arthritis, who, prior to joining a group, always refused to join in any form of physical activity, elected to play a flower in a dramatherapy session. Although she did not leave her chair, her movements became more flexible and expressive as the flower slowly opened. It grew larger and larger and she 'grew' with it.)

Emotional aims and objectives

1. To experience expressing a range of emotions through the creative medium.
2. To do this by using specifically dramatic kinds of media: that is, to explore relationships among people within an imaginative framework which preserves the truthful nature of the emotional experiences involved. (For example, a story about a bad-tempered dwarf allowed an elderly man to inhabit his own resentment against the people whose job it was to care for him. Looking back on his experience in the dwarf's role, he was able to recognize his own grumpiness and, by also rediscovering his sense of humour, he looked on himself with new eyes. There was a consequent improvement in his relationships with his carers.)
3. To maintain and extend sensory perceptions as links with emotional life. (For example, a group were given a variety of large pieces of material which they were then asked to feel — to stroke, to stretch, to fold, to hold against the skin. From these tactile sensations, they went on to describe characters: what kind of climate, household and country would they live in? What scents would accompany different life events in which they took part? How would these materials, environments, scents and so on connect particular emotions they might feel?) This last is an example of the intimate connection our imagination makes between physical and bodily experience and emotional life.

I have listed the main aims and objectives of this adaptation of the creative expressive model, but for every individual group there will be other things to be borne in mind which are to do with that particular group and might not apply elsewhere. Only when you are planning your group will you be able to decide precisely what you are aiming for.

How does working with elderly people differ from working with other client groups?

At the theorectical level, different kinds of groups operate in the same way. Practically speaking, however, there are bound to be some important differences. For instance, when working with groups of elderly people from wards or day rooms, it is a good idea for the group leaders actually to collect each person, rather than asking them to make their own way to the room where the group is to be held, especially if there are any semi- or non-ambulant people.

This gives care staff an opportunity to draw attention to any new problems that may have arisen as a result of a patient's or client's physical disability: for example, how they may need to sit or stand in order to be comfortable. More importantly, however, it helps the client and group leader to establish a physical link. If the client trusts the leader to assist them to the group, they will trust the leader within the group itself if and when they need to move about during group time.

Physical limitations require a high degree of trust on the part of the person who has to live with them; people ought to be able to look to the leader for a degree of awareness of things that others can do but *they* cannot, and which they will need special help with, should the occasion arise. To have been assisted or accompanied to the group lays the foundation for this kind of physical security, without which there may not be enough peace of mind for any real participation in what the group is actually doing.

Although the activities involved in dramatherapy may be similar in the case of different kinds of groups, the ways that they are carried out may differ. For example, another group may kneel or sit on the floor or on bean bags in order to paint a large shared picture, but elderly clients may need different seating arrangements and adapted equipment. Ted Wharam, a dramatherapist, in conversation with the author, suggested tying brushes to poles to enable painting on a large sheet of paper placed on the floor. An alternative may be to have the paper on a table and use decorating or paste brushes with paints in large cans or mixed in bowls. Thus the same kind of picture is painted in a different way: what is adapted is the technique, rather than the activity itself. (By the way, it is better to improvise your instruments out of whatever is handy, rather than using utensils obviously designed for children and then coping with all the responses to these.)

Instructions should be given clearly, if possible in several ways at once, as some members may find them more difficult to hear, or see or understand, than others. For example, a flip chart and board, using large, clear print, may be used for instructions which are written out beforehand. A pair of leaders stationed in different parts of the room can make announcements one after the other, using exactly the same words. This has the advantage of reassuring those who miss the first announcement. For clarity it also helps to have different kinds of voice ranges. Announcements delivered from more than one direction have more chance of reaching those with restricted hearing. It is up to the leaders to make sure that they can be seen as well as heard.

When working among the elderly we should expect that the actual *range* of physical abilities will be wider than it may be among other groups. Not all elderly people are in wheelchairs; some may attend keep-fit classes. Nor, of course, is every group member confused. Activities must be planned with the whole range of people in mind; it is very easy to fascinate and challenge some, while boring others. The activities should be planned to be flexible enough to engage everyone at the same time.

EXPLORING OUR ATTITUDES TO OLD AGE

Perhaps we have fixed ideas about what it is to be elderly, or perhaps we have not. Perhaps — and this is more likely — we have fixed ideas and do not know we have them. This is because there is a tendency, when it comes to guessing about how other people feel, to be rather wide of the mark. For one thing, we cannot avoid judging the situation in terms of the one we are in ourselves. This can be misleading, because we just cannot know all the factors involved and tend either to underestimate the difference between us and them or to imagine it to be greater than it is. For another thing, we can only imagine other people's lives according to the way we perceive our own, and this always blurs our vision: we are wearing the wrong spectacles and, if we attempt to borrow theirs, we are going to find it even harder to focus. So there is really no alternative to letting them tell us, or actively encouraging them to tell us, what it is like.

This means that, whether or not we ourselves are elderly, our understanding of what being elderly means will never become fixed. It will always be changing in the light of new evidence as we adjust our ideas and expectations of other people according to the things we would never have known unless they had revealed them to us, often in exchange for our willingness to be seen by them as the people we are. Fixed ideas are extremely powerful: they influence the way we interpret everything that happens. To see someone always in the same way, adhering always to the received guidelines, is to treat them in a very extreme way indeed; it is to depersonate a person before you have even met them. It does not matter if your preconceived idea is mild and non-judgemental; it is a conclusion already drawn, and drawn prematurely. It does not matter if it is only the outline of a particular kind of person; it will always affect the details as we try to confirm the correctness of our outline.

This is particularly so if we know someone very well who is elderly — or if we are elderly ourselves. In both these cases we are particularly prone to 'knowing what it is all about'. The surer we are that we do know, the more dangerous we can be. It is better to be open-minded and willing to add to our store of understanding and skill. Groupwork with people of all ages depends on human relationships and interactions. These relationships can be affected and influenced by conscious and unconscious prejudices, stereotyping and attitudes. Before undertaking groupwork with the elderly it is useful to unearth some of our attitudes which may affect our relationship with the client group.

Set aside some time to complete the following exercises. Be prepared to accept the first words or images that surface as useful indications of barriers that may be present between you and the group members.

Exercise 1

The following visualizations are designed for use when you are in a relaxed state. Record them onto tape, remember or ask someone to read them to you.

Imagine that you are in a large park on a bright, sunny day. Flowers are in bloom; the grass is green and newly mowed. You walk along the path feeling happy, smiling at the people you meet. You notice two elderly people sitting on a bench. How old are they? How are they dressed?

They smile at you and invite you to sit with them. You immediately form an idea about why they want you to sit with them. What is your idea? You sit with them for a while and talk. What do you talk about?

After some time you leave and continue your walk. Approaching you is a young person pushing a pushchair. You stop and talk to the young person. How do you interact with them? You turn your attention to the child in the pushchair and say a few words. The child smiles and you continue with the interaction. You part company and continue your walk.

Approaching you, you see a middle-aged person pushing a wheelchair with a person in their early seventies seated comfortably and enjoying the sunshine. You stop and speak to them in turn. What order have you chosen? What do you talk to them about?

You say good-bye and walk towards a shady place under a tree. You sit on the grass and rest your back against the tree. You feel comfortable here and start to reflect on the interactions you have engaged in.

How did age and gender influence your expectations of other people and the content and tone of the conversation? Are there any of your approaches you would like to change? If so, imagine yourself repeating the meeting, but with the changes you would like to make. What difference do these changes make?

Return to an alert state and reflect on the way your attitudes could affect interactions with clients.

Now imagine that you are in a large house. It is a home for an extended family of grandparents, parents and children. How do the furnishings, ornaments and decoration reflect the age ranges of the people who live here?

You are a friend of the family and have agreed to organize a joint surprise birthday party for one of the grandparents who will be 90 and a child who will be celebrating their fifth birthday. What needs do you anticipate they will have? How do you plan to decorate the house for the party?

The first shop you visit is a gift shop where you choose wrapping paper and other paper items. The next shop is a baker's, where you select the birthday cakes. What have you considered in making your choices?

When you reach the supermarket, you start to fill your trolley with goods, some specifically for the child and some for the 89-year-old. As you choose each item, reflect on your choices. How are your selections influenced by the genders you have given the two people and by their ages? There will be some items you select for both of them. What consideration influenced these choices?

Give yourself plenty of time to go round the shop. Become aware, too, of things you reject and why you reject them. End the visualization and reflect on your attitudes.

Exercise 2

Complete the following sentences.

People are old when they ______________________

____

People over 50 are approaching ________________

____

Getting a pension book means __________________

____

People over 60 miss __________________________

____

The major disadvantage of being over 65 is _______

____

When people reach 70 it is unwise to ____________

____

When people are in their seventies, the most exciting thing that can happen to them is ______________

____

The most distressing aspect of old age is _________

____

Each person over 80 is a unique individual, but _____

____

Exercise 3

Have a large sheet of paper and use different coloured felt-tipped pens. Allow ten minutes.

1. Write as many proverbs and sayings as you can think of which concern old age. For example: You can't teach an old dog new tricks; There's life in the old dog yet; Youth and age don't mix; Dirty old man.
2. Paraphrase or sketch images of any advertising which focuses on growing old, such as anti-wrinkle creams, hair colourings or vitamin supplements.

When you have completed the first list, read it through and reflect on how these sayings can influence our attitudes to our clients. For example, have you focused on the external signs of ageing? How does this cause you to react to the way your clients look? Are your sayings more slanted towards the life journey? Are there ways you could expand some of these into group exercises? For example, the saying 'over the hill' can be illustrated further. Draw the hill. What was the journey over the hill like? What is ahead?

Be honest in your reflections. It is sometimes tempting to deny old age. Maybe your second list denies some aspects of growing old. Reflect on how these denials may affect the way you prepare and execute group activities.

It is sometimes helpful to repeat this exercise during the group life and gauge how your attitudes are being changed or shaped by group members.

Exercise 4

You need different coloured felt-tipped pens and a large sheet of paper. Close your eyes and think back to when you were a child and read or listened to fairy stories. Recall these stories. Now write the names of the old people you remember from these stories. When you have written as many names as you can, read them and write their associated characteristics by each in turn.

How are these characteristics influenced by their age? What received ideas did you get from these stories? How have they influenced your attitude?

It may also be useful to return to the sheet and review it in relation to gender. In English we have more words about old women that are designed to be derogatory than we have about old men: for example, hag, crone and 'old bag' always refer to a woman. Redefine some or all of these terms for yourself (crones and hags hold much wisdom).

The same exercise may also be undertaken in reference to culture and race. People from other lands are ofen defined as wicked or barbaric.

The above exercises should help to bring unhelpful attitudes to the fore. Once we are aware of these, we can start to change them.

WHY CHOOSE TO RUN A CREATIVE GROUP?

Before starting to run groups it is very helpful to have a clear idea about why we want to run these groups in particular. The following exercise will help you to clarify your ideas.

Imagine undertaking the group as going on a journey. See yourself as a traveller. Before you start your journey, think about the strengths you already have to help you on your way. These may include training, a good imagination or being good at planning. Make youself a list.

Now imagine yourself at a crossroads. Draw the crossroads. There may be many roads to choose from. Mark one of them 'creative groupwork'. Think of other types of groups and put the names by the roads. On the paper, write in short sentences or single words the reasons why you have chosen this road and rejected the others. (You may not have totally rejected them but, for the moment, they are not your chosen option.) Reflect on what you have written.

Now imagine that a group of unknown people have gathered. They think you have chosen the wrong road. Why do they have this view; what are their criticisms? Write them on another sheet of paper. What do you reply? When you have satisfied yourself that you have finished answering, write a short statement about why you will continue on your way.

Now think about the people you will take with you (co-leaders and participants). Write a letter to them about this exciting journey. Imagine the greatest obstacle and how you will overcome it. Finally, think of other items or qualities that you will need for the journey and how you may obtain them.

It is often useful to keep a record of your journey in a log book and to add to the story each week. You will then have your own creative journal.

POINTS TO CONSIDER BEFORE STARTING CREATIVE GROUPWORK

Co-leaders

Co-leaders are essential for the many roles that will be needed during the group time. It is essential that you can communicate well with your co-leaders:

1. Know each other well enough to be able to take constructive criticism from each other.
2. Define what the tasks are that you will each undertake during the group time.
3. Plan the group for times when you know you will all be available.
4. Chart absences for holidays, study leave and so on before you begin the group. If there are only two leaders, decide whether someone else will substitute for the absent person.
5. Ensure that you all mean the same when you talk about 'creative groupwork'. For example, if one person means knitting and the other means dance and movement, planning will be fraught with difficulties.
6. Set aside a defined time for meeting to plan and evaluate.
7. Ensure that you agree on the aims of the group.

Other workers

1. Do other people know the aims of the group?
2. Is everyone aware of group times and the people who attend the group?
3. Do people know how to refer people?
4. Do you have a referral form for general distribution or other systems?
5. Think of different ways to inform people about the group.

When you feel confident, offer short talks, seminars and care studies to other groups of workers. Cover the following points:

1. How will the group fit into a care programme approach?
2. How will you communicate with key workers?
3. Will you communicate directly with general practitioners or via another agency?
4. Will people continue to attend on discharge? How will this be arranged?
5. How will you communicate with community care workers?

6 How will you communicate with relatives?

7 Find out who will advise you on the protocol and systems for audit and research.

The venue

1 Spend time on finding the right venue. This should not be a room that most group participants use as a daily sitting room. It is better to establish a separate venue so that group time is clearly defined by leaving and entering.

2 Ensure that the group happens in the same room each session.

THE STRUCTURE OF A GROUP

The length of a group session should be considered in relation to the concentration spans of the participants but generally should not be longer than an hour and a half or shorter than half an hour, in order to allow development and maximum focus. Careful consideration should be given to components of the group structure so that they form a coherent whole.

The warm-up

This should take a quarter of the total group time. The main purposes are:

1 to establish or re-establish participants as a group;

2 to tone up the body, voice and imagination; and

3 to stimulate interest and involvement.

The main activity

This should take about half the total group time. The main activity's purposes are:

1 to engage the mind, body and imagination in an artistic union;

2 to promote active expansion of creative impulses;

3 to allow expression of feeling through the dramatic medium;

4 to provide a safe environment for new experiences; and

5 to allow participants to create as an individual and as part of a group.

The closure

This phase aims:

1 to allow time for reflection;

2 to allow participants to 'wind down';

3 to say goodbye to other group members; and

4 to leave the group as an individual.

The following is an example of a one-hour group.

Warm-up	(15 minutes)
Equipment	A4 sheets of card and sheets of paper, coloured felt pens.

Participants are seated around a table. The group leader distributes card and pens. Each person writes their name on the card in large print. In turn they hold up the cards for other to see and say their name. This activity is repeated, but this time participants add short details of a hobby or interest they have now or have enjoyed in the past. They provide a brief description of the interest or hobby as if they are experts providing guidelines for people who would like to take up the hobby themselves. Each person then performs a short mime, using hands only, of their interest or hobby. The others ask questions and the 'expert' replies. The mime is then repeated, slightly amplified. Everyone shakes their hands and arms to loosen them. Small shoulder movements are added, with shoulders moved gently up and down. Now that hands, arms and shoulders have been warmed up, participants repeat their mime with enlarged movements.

Main activity (30 minutes)

The ideas of experts, interests and hobbies have now been introduced. Now each person thinks of a fictional person who is an expert: for example, Sherlock Holmes as an expert detective, Scrooge as an expert miser or King Arthur as an expert knight. On the other side of their cards each person writes the name of the fictional character. In turn each person says a few words about their character's area of expertise.

After each person has provided this description, everyone shows the other group members a brief mime of the character engaged in performing an action within their area of expertise. Following this they again shake their arms and hands and relax their shoulders by making shrugging movements. The group leader then encourages participants to sit upright, to move into the posture of a person who is proud of their achievements. The group are then asked to think how their characters might talk about their particular skills. They are asked to adjust their posture to move into an attitude that the character might adopt in order to praise themselves. Each person says a few words as the character. For example, Sherlock Holmes could say, "I am a brilliant detective. I have solved the most complex and difficult of crimes." The other characters may make brief comments, such as "That was very clever" or "I really do admire your skill."

When everyone has spoken they relax their postures. Large sheets of paper and pens are issued to participants. Each person draws an award for their character. When the pictures are completed, each person shows the other participants the award they have drawn. Following this, everyone decides which actions from their own lives they recall with pride.

The group ends with each group member saying good-bye to the others by shaking their hands and telling them something they like about them.

This group has focused on posture, upper body flexibility and positive self-image, through the characters and then directly relating to group members themselves. Small dramas have been created while participants have remained seated. It is also possible to carry on all of the activity if one or two members lose concentration or need to leave for any reason.

PREPARING FOR THE GROUP: A CHECKLIST

The venue

- Is it available?
- Temperature
- Is everything safe?
- Will there be any distracting noise from outside?
- Is the group space private?
- Is furniture arranged in order to provide access to and from toilets?
- Are other staff aware that a group will be taking place?

The equipment

- Is it safe?
- Is it all in working order?
- Do you have everything you need?
- Is back-up material readily available?

The group members

- Can everyone stay for the duration of the group?
- Does everyone have everything they need?
- Has anyone just been involved in a stressful interview or situation?
- Are all the staff involved with the group aware of any changes in physical abilities of group members?

It is helpful to prepare your own checklist which is specific to your group members and environment.

Let us look at each heading in more detail.

The venue

Is it available?

It is worth taking the time to check before each group even though a block booking may have been made. Very often you will need to take into account the times when decorating or repairs are scheduled or when other bookings have been made.

Temperature

As well as the actual temperature in the room this should include checking that temperature gauges on radiators are working, that windows can be opened or closed and that any draughts can be safely blocked. It is also advisable to ensure that group members bring cardigans, shawls or jackets that can be added to their attire without disruption to the group activity.

Safety

Check furniture, equipment, access and floor coverings. Group members may be moving in an unfamiliar manner and hazards may become more pronounced.

Noise

It is vitally important to check for any unwanted noise that may occur during the group and to prevent this as a source of disruption. This may include cleaning, repair work, people en route to a meeting, functions, groups of visitors or replacing furniture.

As a rule, notices asking for silence do not work; in fact, people reading them out loud to communicate the message to others may add to noise levels. It is usually better to make verbal requests in advance, if possible, or to ask someone not involved in the group to take charge of noise prevention. If none of these options is viable, establish in advance which facilitator will leave to deal with the disruption. It is helpful to be proactive rather than reactive.

Privacy

For group members to feel safe, a private and uninterrupted environment is essential. Making sure that people not involved in the group do not enter the room while the group is in progress is an obvious precaution, but it is also important to ensure that group activities cannot be observed in other ways. It is inhibiting to suddenly realize that one has an audience peering through a glass door panel or window.

'DO NOT DISTURB' signs tend to be ineffective; it is usually more helpful to make a list of people who may enter and write to them before starting the series of groups and to follow this up with verbal reminders.

Other staff — transport and ambulance workers, and voluntary staff who bring sweet trollies, for example — will appreciate prior notice.

Access

We tend to think of groups taking place with members sitting in a circle. There are very good reasons for this: circular arrangement of seating enables everyone to see everyone else, verbal communication can be easier and the circle has strong symbolic meanings of unity, equality and trust. However, with this particular client group, it may be more practical to work in other ways and to construct the initial seating arrangements to facilitate easy access to toilets, leaving adequate space between chairs for people to walk or be transported through. Again, careful consideration before the group will help to prevent unnecessary disruptions during the group.

Other staff

Some of the matters relating to other staff have been dealt with under the heading of privacy, but there are some other important issues to consider. Creative groupwork can be noisy. For example, if people are engaged in making sounds, some exercises include sounds to represent the weather and these can be misinterpreted as sounds of distress if people are not aware that drama is taking place.

It can be annoying for staff from other departments to visit areas to make appointments or to interview clients only to be told they are engaged in groupwork and cannot be disturbed. Therefore, as mentioned earlier, make the times and days of the group as widely known as possible.

The equipment

Is it safe?

Safety factors are always important but, because the group members may have slower reactions and responses, or some degree of confusion, we do need to be extra vigilant. Check items like trailing leads from electrical equipment and ensure that they are not in places where they can cause people to trip or fall over. If any electrical equipment is supplied from home or a place other than the group base, make sure that it is checked by an electrician before it is used. Check that furniture with sharp edges, for example tables, is not positioned near spaces to be used for movement.

It is useful to brainstorm all the possible danger presented by anything in the group room. This can be fun if taken to ludicrous extremes, but can reveal some relevant but not immediately obvious dangers. This could also be an exercise for group members to do, as it may add different perspectives.

Is it all in working order?

All equipment for use in any group should be checked to make sure it is in working order. This applies to all forms of groupwork but, again, specific considerations do apply to this area of work. For example, with younger people a felt-tip pen that has run out can be replaced by taking another from the container in a matter of seconds. These groups may have members who are less agile. This task will probably take longer, which will break concentration or cause dependency on leaders to perform the task for them. Time can be wasted in identifying whether more pressure from pen to paper is required before it is realized that the pen is not working. This can lead to a sense of frustration and an unwillingness to try again with a replacement.

It is helpful to practise each exercise in advance of the group to check that even simple items will work in the way you intend them to. For example, will the card actually fold; are the scissors sharp enough to cut the fabric you intend to use; are the items you intend to use for music work complete? Does the gong have the correct stick to provide sound? A golden rule is: never use anything for the first time in the group situation.

Do you have everything you need?

Create equipment lists as you plan the group and start to collect equipment days rather than hours before the group time. This will provide the chance to rework some exercises if the equipment you need is not available. As mentioned above, a practice run of each exercise will highlight any omissions.

Is back-up material readily available?

As quite a few of the exercises in this book, particularly in the puppet and mask section, require a range of equipment, it is sometimes difficult to anticipate exactly what group members may need to create exactly the effect they want to achieve. While it may not always be possible to meet their requirements, a well catalogued collection of equipment may enable you to provide an acceptable substitute. It is essential that additional material is easy to find. It is helpful if it is stored in stackable containers with the contents marked clearly on the outside of the box. If your store cupboard is not in the same place as the venue for the group, it is sometimes helpful to place them on a trolley and take them into the group.

The group members

As has already been indicated, it is helpful for the people who will be leading the group to be involved in the arrival stage. This also gives them time for checking that group members have everything they need with them. Items such as spectacles and other small but essential objects can be forgotten and cause great distress when they are missed.

In addition to checking whether any changes have taken place in the group members' emotional and physical health between groups, it is advisable to find out if they have received any other changes to treatments or care regimes on the day of the group. Having this information can help the group leader to broach the subject, if appropriate, or to be aware that the client's reactions to the group activity may be influenced by immediately prior events.

Can everyone stay for the duration of the group?

There are a host of reasons why even the most committed group members (or indeed, leaders) may have to leave a group before the time planned to close the session. While pre-planning can avoid this happening frequently, it is sometimes unavoidable. For example, people may need to attend specific events, such as weddings, funerals or retirement functions, or appointments with dentists, doctors or solicitors. People may not want to miss the group, so be adaptable. This may require some reorganization of group activities to allow for departure at an appropriate stage: that is, not in the middle of an improvisation or story-telling activity.

Does everyone have everything they need?

In addition to the considerations relating to equipment which are outlined above, group leaders do also need to think about needs that individual group members may have. Items such as spectacles are not used exclusively by people of this age group, but it may take them longer to go and fetch them from another area. Leaving the group to collect items will be disruptive and cause a lapse of concentration which may be difficult to regain. Be attentive to needs people may have on specific days. Provide tissues if people have colds, footstools or rests if people need to elevate legs and feet for medical reasons, or water if people have to take medication such as antibiotics at set times. Taking the time and trouble to find out or notice these needs before you start can eliminate frustration or disruption during the group.

Has anyone just been involved in a stressful interview or situation?

Groups do not function in isolation from the rest of life. If members have been involved in anxiety-provoking situations then this anxiety will need to be acknowledged by the group leaders, perhaps by speaking to the individual before the group and being aware that the group activity may allow them to express their worries. It is essential to allow people to make the choice about whether they do want to share information with others. Anxieties can sometimes be given emotional expression through the dramatic medium and do not need to be expressed in a direct manner. For example, a particular situation may be explored during a story-telling session and some resolutions discovered by the character within this fictional scenario.

Being aware of changes in physical abilities

These may occur through trauma or ill-health. The importance of networking has already been stressed. To maintain safe practice, maintain regular contact with other care staff.

Many care workers will already be very familiar with items contained in this section on preparation — and may be able to add to the list! Preparing practically for the group is essential, but psychological preparation is of equal importance. Working with a checklist allows the mind to focus on the group members in a way that allows you to know where you have got to in the process of designing the group. It also helps you to work methodically and at your own speed, knowing that when you come to the end of the list you will be more or less ready to start — not only practically, but in the right frame of mind.

Preparing a tool box for creative work

Creative groupwork does not demand a large outlay for equipment. It is often better to adapt easily available items than to buy expensive goods that people may be apprehensive about using. For example, new musical instruments may cause fears about a lack of musical expertise and people will be reluctant to experiment with them to produce sound. It is often helpful to start a small collection of useful items and allow it to grow, rather than trying to obtain everything at once. Such a collection will include the following:

- Different sizes of paper. (It is often worth contacting health promotion units and other health organizations for out-of-date posters. The blank sides are ideal for art work and you will get a variety of sizes.)
- Art materials: felt-tip pens; paints and crayons; scissors.
- Large pieces of fabric with different textures.
- Tins and jars to fill with items such as dried peas, for sound work.
- Large sticks (old mop or broom handles are ideal and can be painted or varnished).
- Nytrim (in different colours). This is a craft material made from shredded nylon remnants which can be obtained from most handicraft specialist catalogues.
- Fabric scraps, lace, fabric flowers.
- Boxes of different sizes.
- Plastic bowls.
- Picture postcards.
- Hats.

As you start to run the groups you will become adept at seeing everyday objects in a new light and adapting them for creative purposes in the group.

Getting down to work

Here are some notes for the leader about things to be borne in mind in the running of every session. First of all, always be aware of the actual physical circumstances of the members of the group. How mobile are they? How well can they use their limbs? What about sight and hearing? These may, for instance, be limitations which may affect the whole group and govern the parameters of any activity you undertake.

Make sure your practice is safe.

People are usually self-conscious about doing things in front of other people. When they get interested in what is going on, this tends to disappear, or at least becomes less noticeable. Try to be confident yourself, from the very beginning.

Never put ideas into people's minds which will tell them what to expect, saying, for example, "You may find this silly but perhaps you'd like to..." or "Perhaps you'll find this difficult, but...". Do not tell people how they will feel; do not tell them it is going to be fun; let them discover their own fun for themselves.

Tailor your approach to the age and situation of the group; do not talk to adults as if they were children. (Elderly people in particular react unfavourably to people who say, "Let's pretend...", "Would it be fun to...?" and so on.) Try to say as clearly as possible what you want the group to do. Be assured rather than tentative, sensitive rather than apologetic. Let group members know from the beginning that you know exactly what you are doing, so that they will be keen on finding out what it is about for themselves.

There is no need for everbody to do everything as if it were a round game, a game in which all, in turn, make a contribution. This kind of procedure has been deliberately avoided in all the activities which follow, which have been arranged so that individual people can either join in or hold back without spoiling the activity. If someone opts out at the beginning and wants to join in later, there is nothing to stop them doing so.

Reminiscence theatre and therapy are not covered in this book as they are well documented elsewhere, and are a different kind of activity with a different purpose. Information about useful books and organizations can be found at the back of this manual.

ASSESSMENT, RECORDING, EVALUATION AND SUPERVISION

Assessment

The assessment procedures must be carried out in a careful and methodical way. The assessment forms provided below (pages 32–50) can be adapted for the needs of a particular group or setting. The assessment interview fulfils several purposes:

1. It makes the first contact between the group leader and potential group participants and thus can be a useful 'ice breaker'. (It can be very frightening to attend your first group, as a leader or participant, without knowing anyone in the room.)
2. It can serve to clarify the aims of the participant and group leader, which may differ from the aims of the referrer.
3. Anxieties that the participant may have can be discussed directly with the group leader, rather than with someone else who may themselves have anxieties about creative work.

Sometimes people have huge anxieties about establishing and carrying out assessment procedures. Somewhere in the back of their minds is a criticizing voice which says that they should be able to work with everyone. This can result in very large groups, containing people with widely different needs and abilities, mostly unknown to the facilitator, who do not want to be activated or engaged in groupwork of any kind. This situation is made even worse if the facilitator has entered their sitting room to struggle to motivate them.

The assessment is not intended to reject or exclude people who may provide a challenge or who do have extra special needs. It is there to ensure that realistic aims can be set and that it is possible for the client to benefit, in some way, from the group. Explain the assessment procedure to other staff before you start, and maybe enlist their help, but do rely on your own judgement about the number of people you can have in the group and who you feel will be most helped by attending.

Recording

Again, the assessment form outlined can be adapted for different settings. Complete the group session form as soon as possible after the end of the group, as perceptions start to become faulty after even a short time. Set aside at least half an hour immediately after the group for reflecting with your co-leaders. Focus on your practice as leaders, the aims of the group and any unexpected adaptations you made, and write down any points that you want to develop in the next session.

This is also the time for entering notes into any other records you have agreed to write.

Evaluation

These forms (see page 50 for an example) should be completed at agreed intervals but not less frequently than one month. You may also agree to produce another form for completion with key workers so that you can assess the kind of improvements that the groupwork is producing outside the group.

Supervision

Supervision is an essential component of good practice which allows us to reflect on and improve the quality of our work. The role of a supervisor is to provide support, to help to develop ideas and to provide an environment where an overview of the group can be taken in an objective way. Sometimes we can sense a difficulty we are having with a particular client but we are unsure why we are experiencing this. A supervisor can help us to unravel these feelings and enable us to perform more effectively.

Ideally, the supervisor for a creative group should be an arts therapist but, if this is not possible, a suitable person trained in groupwork could provide the same kind of support. The British Association for Dramatherapists publishes a list of trained supervisors. The association's address is at the back of this manual.

ASSESSMENT FORM

Date

Name

Date of birth

Address

Record number

Telephone

Registered medical officer (Consultant/General practitioner)

Medical conditions

Medication

Special precautions (eg. for diabetes, epilepsy)

Specific signs and symptoms (any that the group leader may need to be aware of for immediate action, eg. signs and symptoms of angina, diabetic reactions, asthmatic conditions, medication side-effects)

Physical limitations/disabilities

Living circumstances

Reason for attendance/residency at (insert name of centre/hospital)

PHYSICAL MOVEMENT RANGE

		Small	Medium	Large
Right UPPER body	Head			
	Shoulder			
	Arm			
	Hand			
Left UPPER body	Head			
	Shoulder			
	Arm			
	Hand			
	Trunk			
	Waist			
	Hips			
	Pelvis			
Right LOWER body	Leg			
	Thigh			
	Knee			
	Ankle			
	Foot			
Left LOWER body	Leg			
	Thigh			
	Knee			
	Ankle			
	Foot			

ATTITUDE TO GROUPWORK

Movement

Drama

Art

Emotions

Other people

Client's aims (sentence completion)

I will join the group because

What I might achieve is

My major contribution to a group will be

My worries about joining a group are

HOBBIES/MAJOR INTERESTS

Past

Present

Other agencies involved

1

2

3

Summary and agreed aims of client and group leader

Agreed aims

1

2

3

ASSESSMENT FORM

Date *2 February 1996*

Name *John Fairchild*

Date of birth *1/6/1927*

Address *The Hollies*
6 Spindle Road
Woodtown
Countryshire

Record number *16892 10/6*

Telephone *1234 86868*

Registered medical officer (Consultant/General practitioner)

Dr Hope — Consultant psychiatrist

Dr Jindel — General practitioner

Medical conditions

Cancer prostate — diagnosed three months ago.

Medication

Paroxetine 20 mg mane/

cyproterone acetate 100 mg once daily, morning.

Special precautions (eg. for diabetes, epilepsy)

None

Specific signs and symptoms (any that the group leader may need to be aware of for immediate action, eg. signs and symptoms of angina, diabetic reactions, asthmatic conditions, medication side-effects)

None, prostate cancer being treated with medication.

Physical limitations/disabilities

Sometimes needs to make frequent visits to toilet.

Living circumstances

Lives with wife and daughter in own house.

Reason for attendance/residency at (insert name of centre/hospital)

Beeches Day Hospital. Anxiety, panic attacks.

PHYSICAL MOVEMENT RANGE

		Small	Medium	Large
Right UPPER body	Head	✓		
	Shoulder		✓	
	Arm		✓	
	Hand		✓	
Left UPPER body	Head		✓	
	Shoulder		✓	
	Arm		✓	
	Hand		✓	
	Trunk		✓	
	Waist		✓	
	Hips	✓		
	Pelvis	✓		
Right LOWER body	Leg		✓	
	Thigh		✓	
	Knee		✓	
	Ankle		✓	
	Foot		✓	
Left LOWER body	Leg		✓	
	Thigh		✓	
	Knee		✓	
	Ankle		✓	
	Foot		✓	

ATTITUDE TO GROUPWORK

Movement

He used to walk a lot, before he started to have bad panic attacks. Became a bit frightened of going out. "I would like to build up movement again."

Drama

He used to watch television quite a lot. Liked the drama series but does not know if he could do it himself.

Art

Never done any drawing. Has never thought about it as something he could do.

Emotions

Used to keep them to himself, "bottled them up, but talking about how I feel helps."

Other people

Stopped noticing other people when he was very anxious but "I'm just starting to notice them a bit now".

Client's aims (sentence completion)

I will join the group because *I would like to start a bit of movement again. I found the other group I'm in very helpful.*

What I might achieve is *some more self-confidence. Feeling relaxed again.*

My major contribution to a group will be *I've a good sense of humour. It's just starting to surface again.*

My worries about joining a group are *I have out-patient appointments at the general out-patients and might miss some.*

HOBBIES/MAJOR INTERESTS

Past

Walking, breeding dogs

Present

Watching television

Other agencies involved

1. *Jean Reid — one-to-one sessions dealing with anxieties about prostate cancer.*
2. *Katherine Martin — John a participant in anxiety management group.*
3. *Dr Hope — supports John's involvement in group.*

Summary and agreed aims of client and group leader

A 67-year-old man who is attending for three days per week. Retired at the age of 65 from a time-consuming job as a school caretaker. Enjoyed this work but became very tired and tense during the last year. Is keen to join the group and was animated and talkative during the initial interview. Some concerns about the creative work but was reassured that the drama components will not involve learning complicated texts – a worry he expressed towards the end of the interview. Movement assessment done in interview by movement to music.

Agreed aims

1. *To engage in movement to promote relaxation.*
2. *To allow himself to express his feelings in relation to the creative structures.*
3. *To stimulate interest in others and self.*

ASSESSMENT FORM

Date *6 June 1996*

Name *Martha Tindall*

Date of birth *3/5/1918*

Address *6 The Spinney*
Meadow Road
Woodtown
Countryshire

Record number *N/A*

Telephone *1234 98762*

Registered medical officer (Consultant/General practitioner)

Dr Thymore — General practitioner

Medical conditions

None

Medication

None

Special precautions (eg. for diabetes, epilepsy)

None

Specific signs and symptoms (any that the group leader may need to be aware of for immediate action, eg. signs and symptoms of angina, diabetic reactions, asthmatic conditions, medication side-effects)

None

Physical limitations/disabilities

None known

Living circumstances

Lives with friend in own house.

Reason for attendance/residency at (insert name of centre/hospital)

Church social club for social activities for over 65s

PHYSICAL MOVEMENT RANGE

		Small	Medium	Large
Right UPPER body	Head			✓
	Shoulder			✓
	Arm			✓
	Hand			✓
Left UPPER body	Head			✓
	Shoulder			✓
	Arm			✓
	Hand			✓
	Trunk		✓	
	Waist		✓	
	Hips		✓	
	Pelvis		✓	
Right LOWER body	Leg		✓	
	Thigh		✓	
	Knee		✓	
	Ankle		✓	
	Foot		✓	
Left LOWER body	Leg		✓	
	Thigh		✓	
	Knee		✓	
	Ankle		✓	
	Foot		✓	

ATTITUDE TO GROUPWORK

Movement

Goes to quite a few dancing classes, ballroom and sequence dancing, also some tea dances. Enjoys moving.

Drama

Is used to dance but has never done any drama. "I suppose it is quite close."

Art

Never been interested in art, "but if it is in small doses, I can try".

Emotions

"I'm okay. Maybe it is good, sometimes, to have a place to talk over things."

Other people

Gets on well with people but likes to have time to herself sometimes.

Client's aims (sentence completion)

I will join the group because *it will be a new experience and will be a different form of communication.*

What I might achieve is *different types of movement; a chance to see if I do like art.*

My major contribution to a group will be *I can be a good companion.*

My worries about joining a group are *Maybe I won't like the art and will find it too different.*

HOBBIES/MAJOR INTERESTS

Past

Walking, reading novels, patchwork, dancing

Present

Walking, reading novels, patchwork, dancing

Other agencies involved

1. *Letter to Dr Thymore to outline aims of group and to inform him Miss Tindall will be joining.*
2.
3.

Summary and agreed aims of client and group leader

Miss Tindall is a very active woman with a wide variety of interests in social and physical areas of her life. During the initial interview the aims of the group have been outlined to her and she seems to understand the differences between this group and the other activities she is involved in.

Agreed aims

1. *To explore her and others' attitudes to old age within a structured activity.*
2. *To extend her creative impulses.*
3. *To explore her needs for her own space and develop ways of creating this within creative structures.*

ASSESSMENT FORM

Date *1 February 1996*

Name *Elizabeth Jenkyns (likes to be called Betty)*

Date of birth *6/1/1920*

Record number *1246810/2*

Address *65 Bankfield Road*
Woodtown
Countryshire

Telephone *None, neighbour Mrs Rowan 1234 56789*

Registered medical officer (Consultant/General practitioner)

Dr Khan — Consultant psychiatrist

Dr Heldon — General practitioner

Medical conditions

Angina — ten years' duration

Medication

Glyceryl/trinitrate, one to two when needed. Nifedipine 10 mg three times daily.

Special precautions (eg. for diabetes, epilepsy)

Attending physiotherapy for recent wrist injury; sprained right wrist after fall in street during snow.

Specific signs and symptoms (any that the group leader may need to be aware of for immediate action, eg. signs and symptoms of angina, diabetic reactions, asthmatic conditions, medication side-effects)

Angina — Mrs Jenkyns is familiar with pains that signal onset. Likes to keep her handbag near her to reach glyceryl/trinitrate.

Physical limitations/disabilities

Caution with use of right wrist.

Living circumstances

Living alone in council house. Visited by son, three times a week; neighbours visit daily.

Reason for attendance/residency at (insert name of centre/hospital)

Beeches Day Hospital, Mental Health Unit. Depression coupled with prolonged grief reaction to husband's death ten years ago.

PHYSICAL MOVEMENT RANGE

		Small	Medium	Large
Right UPPER body	Head		✓	
	Shoulder		✓	
	Arm	✓ (Limited owing to		
	Hand	✓ recent injury)		
Left UPPER body	Head		✓	
	Shoulder		✓	
	Arm		✓	
	Hand		✓	
	Trunk	✓		
	Waist	✓		
	Hips	✓		
	Pelvis	✓		
Right LOWER body	Leg	✓		
	Thigh	✓		
	Knee	✓		
	Ankle	✓		
	Foot	✓		
Left LOWER body	Leg	✓		
	Thigh	✓		
	Knee	✓		
	Ankle	✓		
	Foot	✓		

ATTITUDE TO GROUPWORK

Movement

Worried that this may be too strenuous. Attends keep fit during time at this centre, states that she enjoys this but likes to stay in her chair.

Drama

Slightly anxious; thought she would have to perform as a solo player.

Art

Some worries about her art work being displayed and critizized. Has not done any painting or drawing since school.

Emotions

Thinks they should be kept to oneself. "It's not fair to burden others."

Other people

"I try to get on with other people." Believes that she needs to please others all the time.

Client's aims (sentence completion)

I will join the group because *I would, maybe, like to start mixing with other people again. I only see people who visit me. I used to go out a lot.*

What I might achieve is *saying how I sometimes feel. I always say 'I'm all right.' I'm not used to mixing well now.*

My major contribution to a group will be *a willingness to try new things.*

My worries about joining a group are *that I will have to say a lot and I won't be able to act well.*

HOBBIES/MAJOR INTERESTS

Past

Sewing, knitting, pressing wild flowers

Present

None

Other agencies involved

1 *Physiotherapy - Jane Harris*
2 *Occupational therapy - Thelma Adcock*
3 *Key nurse - Amanda Wilson*
4 *Consultant psychiatrist - Dr Kahn*
5 *Care programme co-ordinator–social worker — Allan Irwin*

Agreed aims

1 *Jane Harris seen — explained wrist exercises — some caution with movement.*
2 *Thelma Adcock — home assessment completed. No problems isolated.*
3 *Amanda Wilson — feels that involvement in group will encourage communication.*
4 *Dr Kahn — also feels that involvement in group will encourage communication.*
5 *Allan Irwin — next meeting of care team, 6 March at 2.30pm. Group leaders to be invited and to discuss agreed aims of client and group leader.*

HOBBIES/MAJOR INTERESTS

Summary and agreed aims of client and group leader

A 75-year-old lady who has been attending the Beeches for six months on a daily basis following discharge from Mental Health Unit, in-patient treatment for 12 weeks for depression and prolonged grief reaction. Key nurse — Amanda Wilson — is seeing her on an individual basis to encourage her to express her grief; may consider referral to therapist but reports that she is starting to talk about how much she misses her husband.

A rather solitary woman who speaks in a soft, rather hesitant way but makes appropriate eye contact. Body is almost motionless during conversation. Movement range assessed during keep-fit class, run by occupational therapy helper.

Initially very worried about becoming involved in creative groupwork. Tended to view this as competitive and feared that her efforts would be judged. I was able to reassure her on these points and explained the aims of the group.

Agreed aims

1. *To extend communication skills and range.*
2. *To engage in activities with an emphasis on self-esteem rather than usual emphasis on pleasing others.*
3. *To extend range of perceptions of the environment. Currently focused on her immediate home.*
4. *To extend movement ranges.*

GROUP SESSION FORM

Date **Session number**

Present

Absent (and why)

Activity

Aims

Were aims met?

MONTHLY EVALUATION FORM

Name **Record number**

Date of birth

Physical		No change	Some change	Marked change	Do not know
Upper body	Flexibility				
	Recognition				
	Awareness				
	Movements in place				
	Comments				
Trunk	Flexibility				
	Recognition				
	Awareness				
	Movement				
	Comments				
Lower body	Flexibility				
	Recognition				
	Awareness				
	Movement				
	Comments				
Emotional	Expression				
	Imagination				
	Communication				
	Enjoyment				
	Interaction				
	Comments				

Have the client's stated aims been achieved?

Comments from others not involved in group (other staff, relatives)

PERFORMING AND PERFORMANCE

Before considering a group performance it is essential to be absolutely clear about *why* you are intending to share the created work with people outside the group. Consider the reasons that group leaders might have for presentation of creative groupwork, and the reasons that group members might have for performing. Prepare lists of these and deal with any conflicting motives.

For example, group leaders might want to show colleagues that they have not been wasting time in running the group, while group members might want to share fun with other clients or residents. This represents a possible conflict of reasons for performing: the group leaders want to impress others and show the serious intentions behind their work, while group members want to play and share the experience of a sense of fun they have found in the drama.

Be aware of some of the disadvantages and advantages of performance.

Some disadvantages

1. Performance may be very anxiety provoking.
2. Spontaneity in improvisations may become lost.
3. Rehearsal involves repetition of material. This repetition can create boredom and conflict if group members are not all totally committed to performance.
4. Group members may become doubtful of their own creativity as the reality of playing to an audience comes closer.
5. More skilled members may become frustrated with less able members during the rehearsal period.
6. The absence of any member or members can cause difficulties and resentment.

Some advantages

1. The sharing of creative work with others can be a confirming and validating experience.
2. Performance can unite the group and promote self-sufficiency.
3. Increased confidence about abilities and self-worth.

4 Improved concentration and co-operation.

5 Dramatic ideas and concepts can be explored in greater depth during the rehearsal period.

6 The presence of an audience from outside the group can re-energize a group.

If you decide that performance will be beneficial for everyone involved, there are several important areas to consider.

What to perform

Will the material to be performed be based on work created in previous groups or is it to be created specifically for the performance? Will the drama be an adaptation of an established text or story, or will it be formed from ideas generated by the participants' imagination?

What will be the major concepts or ideas to be conveyed to the audience?

What will be the style and form of the performance? How will the start, middle and end be structured? What will be the first image that the audience will see? How will this prepare them for the style of the performance? It is important to be clear about a careful combination of content and style. As soon as the group has decided upon the content, devise your style: *what* to perform must be very closely linked to *how* to perform within the capabilities of group members. For example, it would obviously be inappropriate to present *Cinderella* in a tragic mode, as a farce or a thriller. However this story could be presented in an imagistic way, as a mixture of comedy and pathos, a melodrama or as a partly narrated and partly performed play. A clearly defined style will unify acting modes and present a coherent form of theatre.

The actor/audience relationship

The audience needs to be present in the players' imaginations from the outset. Awareness of the eventual presence of spectators will help the actors to learn to project communication to them as well as to each other. To make this communication as effective as possible, the following decisions need to be made:

1 Where will the playing area be?

2 How large will it be?

3 What shape will it be? Are sight lines good?

4 How will the play be performed to the audience? Will it

be in the round; will the audience be seated in straight rows, in a horseshoe shape, or a semi-circle?

5 How close to the audience will the actors be?

6 Are the acoustics in the chosen area good? Will the audience be able to hear?

7 Is it best to choose a playing area away from doors in case any latecomers enter the playing area? If this is not possible, plan courses of action to prevent interruption.

8 Will you have an 'off stage' area, or will all the actors remain in view throughout the performance, maybe seated on chairs surrounding the playing area when not directly involved in the action?

Costumes and props

It is useful to keep these to an absolute minimum as they can be fraught with hazards for the inexperienced player. Anxieties about props, in particular, can cause unnecessary delays during the rehearsal period and have been known to ruin an otherwise sound performance by being in the wrong place, faulty or mishandled by an actor owing to performance nerves.

Rehearsal time can often be usefully spent on mime skills, which provide a source of concentration, co-ordination and self-sufficiency, instead of focusing on props.

If you do decide that some costumes and/or props are essential for your production, the following guidelines may be useful:

1 Have the actual costume or prop ready for use in the early rehearsal period. If this is not possible, have substitutes available. For example, movement in a long skirt is different from movement in a shorter one, so if long skirts are produced at a dress rehearsal, it will be too late for adapting movement. Miming with props before they actually appear is usually unhelpful as the actual prop will almost certainly be heavier than expected, of a different shape and less adaptable.

2 Costumes can be representational. Instead of creating a full costume, use one unrestricting item of clothing: for example, a shawl, an apron, a hat or a waistcoat.

3 Use Velcro for fastenings: it causes fewer problems than zips or buttons.

4 Decide on costume details very early in the production planning. Co-ordinate the designs. Be clear about what people will be wearing and keep this the same for every performance. If people wear their everyday clothes, it is sometimes tempting for them to wear what they happen to be wearing that day without taking account of the movement restrictions imposed by tight clothing.

5 Designate one person to be in charge of costumes and props. Make it absolutely clear that this person is in charge and will be responsible for their availability at rehearsal and performance.

6 Be very strict about not accepting the introduction of props towards the end of the rehearsal period. People often have very good ideas about performance-enhancing props near the performance time, but they are equally often confusing and difficult to manage when introduced too late.

Performances can be fun, exciting and very emotionally moving for both the actors and the audience. For the performers it is usually helpful if the performance follows the same format as the group: warm-up, performance and closure. The warm-up and closure should be a mixture of body movement, voice and concentration exercises. Many of these can be found in this manual and other sources are supplied in the Bibliography in Section 3.

SECTION 2

ACTIVITIES

WARM-UPS AND STARTERS

MOVEMENT 1

Focus Head and back flexibility; dramatic movement

Time 10 minutes

Equipment None

Activity

1. Sit in chairs, feet firmly on floor. Check balance.
2. Move trunk and head forwards, to centre and towards back of chair.
3. Repeat three times.
4. Imagine that you are wearing a large, wide-brimmed hat with elaborate trimmings or a top hat. How will wearing this hat affect your head and back posture? You are a very important person. How does this status affect your posture and the way you look at other people?
5. Mime your own way of taking off this hat.
6. You are wearing a very old headscarf or cap. You are cold and feel unimportant. How is your posture affected by this status?
7. Mime unknotting a scarf and folding it.
8. Imagine wearing a favourite hat. How do you feel? Show your posture as if you want to look your best for a photograph.
9. Group leaders or other group members mime taking the photographs.

Adaptations

1. Pose for a group photograph.
2. Have a hat collection and use actual hats.

WARM-UPS AND STARTERS

MOVEMENT 2

Focus Flexibility of feet, legs, hips

Time 10 minutes

Equipment None

Activity

1. Sit well back in your chair.
2. Move your feet into different positions.
3. Imagine the floor is covered with a thick, bouncy covering. Move your feet as if they are bouncing on this surface.
4. Imagine the floor is very sticky and it is hard to move your feet. Move them slowly as if they become more and more difficult to move.
5. Imagine the floor is covered with a thick, soft carpet. Allow your feet to sink into it. Relax. Let the feeling from your feet spread through your whole body.

Adaptations

1. Create more floor surfaces for movement, such as ice, mud, hard pavings or crazy pavings.
2. Play appropriate taped music to enhance movement.
3. Have some people in chairs, others moving around the room.

WARM-UPS AND STARTERS

MOVEMENT 3

Focus Fine and gross movements of hands, arms, shoulders

Time 10 minutes

Equipment Soft light, cushions or pillows

Activity

1. Group members sit well back in their chairs.
2. Each group member has a cushion or pillow on their lap.
3. Place your hands on the cushion or pillow and knead it gently.
4. With your hands make movements like a cat clawing at a cushion.
5. 'Plump up' the cushion with big hand movements.
6. Imagine that you are going to embroider a pattern onto the cover. Thread the needle, slowly and with small, precise movements.
7. Sew with small, neat stitches.
8. Imagine the cushion as a piece of dough and knead it with large movements.
9. Shake your hands and relax.

Adaptations

1. Ask group members about other craft hobbies or interests they have and mime these.
2. Ask what else the cushion could represent and mime suggestions.
3. Work in pairs: sewing, mending, stuffing.

WARM-UPS AND STARTERS

MOVEMENT 4

Focus Leg and knee flexibility

Time 15 minutes

Equipment Ball of thick string or nytrim

Activity

1. In a chair, move your feet two or three inches apart.
2. Move your left leg and foot half an inch from the ground, then replace it on the floor. Move your right leg and foot half an inch from the ground. Put it back down. Repeat two or three times.
3. Leader places string or nytrim in a circle inside the group, near to members' feet.
4. Imagine the space inside the nytrim or string circle as a pool of clear water.
5. Place one foot, toe first, into the water. It is cold. Remove your foot and shake it.
6. Repeat with your other foot.
7. Place one foot into the water. It feels nice. Splash a little. Put your other foot into the pool. Splash about with both feet.
8. Remove your feet and shake them dry.

Adaptations

1. Walk into the pool and paddle.
2. Splash with your hands as well.
3. The pool is frozen. Break the ice with your feet.

WARM-UPS AND STARTERS

MOVEMENT 5

Focus Shoulder and arm flexibility; balance

Time 10 minutes

Equipment None

Activity

1. Shrug your shoulders, then shrug again, bringing your shoulders as near to your ears as possible. Relax and repeat.
2. Lift your left shoulder. Relax. Lift your right shoulder. Relax.
3. Raise your right arm. Relax. Raise your left arm. Relax. Raise your right arm. Relax. Repeat.
4. Shake your arms and hands.
5. Hold your right arm out in front of your body, palm down.
6. Imagine a soft ball balanced on the back of your right arm. Make gentle bouncing movements to move the ball towards your right shoulder. Relax your arm. Bounce the ball on your shoulder. Bounce it to your left shoulder, bounce it on your left shoulder. Raise your left arm. Bounce the ball down your left arm.
7. Relax your arms and shoulders. Shake your hands.
8. Bounce the ball onto the floor.

Adaptations

1. Use imaginary balls of different shapes and sizes, and different movements for each size.
2. In pairs, bounce imaginary balls between you. Add kicking movements.

WARM-UPS AND STARTERS

MOVEMENT 6

Focus Hand, wrist, arm flexibility; relaxation

Time 10 minutes

Equipment None

Activity

1. Shake your hands and fingers.
2. Shake your hands, fingers and wrists.
3. Shake your hands, fingers, wrists and arms.
4. Lean right back in your chair.
5. Relax in your chair.
6. Imagine it is a cold night and you are sitting in a warm room in front of a log fire.
7. Reach your hands out towards the fire to warm them. Relax.
8. A cold draught comes into the room. You fold your arms across your body in reaction.
9. The cold diminishes and you relax again, feeling very comfortable.
10. You warm your hands at the fire again and relax.

Adaptations

1. For a group that likes cats, add: a cat is sitting on your lap. Stroke the cat.
2. For additional movements, add logs to the fire.
3. Add movement for more ambulant group members: pulling curtains, switching on/off lights, stoking the fire.

WARM-UPS AND STARTERS

MOVEMENT 7

Focus Head, trunk, hand and arm movement; flexibility, fine and gross

Time 10 minutes

Equipment None

Activity

1 Group members sit or stand in a row.

2 Move your head slowly to the right and then to the left. Repeat twice.

3 Move your right arm to the front, then your left arm. Repeat twice.

4 You are all in a queue. Which end is the front? It is a bus queue.

5 Look into the distance to see if the bus is coming.

6 Look at your watches.

7 They are always late. Shake your heads and look at your watches again.

8 The bus is coming. Watch it come nearer.

9 It does not look as if it will stop. Put out your arms to signal it to stop.

10 It is full. Shrug your shoulders in reaction to the bus going past you.

11 It is getting cold. Rub your arms and shoulders.

12 The next bus comes. Put your arms out to stop it.

13 Relax in relief as the bus stops.

Adaptations

1 Create different kinds of queues. Add movements.

2 Add conversation between the waiting people.

3 Group members create sounds: wind, rain or footsteps of passers-by.

4 Develop into drama for a main activity.

WARM-UPS AND STARTERS

MOVEMENT 8

Focus Trunk, arm and hand flexibility; using the imagination; large movements

Time 10 minutes

Equipment None

Activity

1. Sit back in your chair.
2. Move forward from the waist. Move back. Move forward again. Check that your balance is safe.
3. Place your feet firmly on the ground.
4. Balanced against your knees is a scrubbing/washing board. Make the movement of rubbing a delicate piece of fabric against the board.
5. Rub a heavy piece of clothing against the board.
6. Rub a heavily stained garment against the board.
7. Put the board to one side.
8. Wring out the washing.
9. Hang it out to dry (sitting or standing).

Adaptations

1. Half of the group creates a rubbing rhythm by clapping their hands. The other half move to the rhythm. Change after five minutes.
2. Work in pairs, with one person on each side of the board.
3. Sit in threes or fours around an imaginary huge tub of water. As a group describe the details of the tub of water. Mime doing some washing in the tub.

WARM-UPS AND STARTERS

MOVEMENT 9

Focus Toning up the arms and hands; increasing flexibility; body awareness

Time 10 minutes

Equipment None

Activity

1. Rub your hands gently together, palms inwards.
2. Change to a soft wringing movement.
3. Rub your hands together as if rubbing on hand cream.
4. Rub your palms together. Part and hold your palms about half an inch apart. Feel the heat generated by the rubbing.
5. Rub your hands again and hold them an inch or so apart. Feel the changes in the energy generated.
6. Find different ways of holding your palms together. Involve your arms and elbows.

Adaptations

1. Add music to suggest different movements.
2. Work with a partner. Feel the energy coming from their palms.
3. Move your palms around face and head to feel different body temperatures.

WARM-UPS AND STARTERS

MOVEMENT 10

Focus Finger flexibility, awareness of sounds, moving bags out of the way

Time 10 minutes

Equipment Participants own handbags, other bags for those without

Activity

1. Sit back in your chair.
2. Place your handbag on your lap.
3. Close your eyes or look away and feel the texture and shape of the bag.
4. Tap your fingers on the surface and feel the difference in contact. Listen for any sound.
5. Place your bag on another part of your lap. Make different sounds. Open your eyes.
6. Imagine your bag is very heavy and move it to another place on your lap.
7. Still imagining that it is very heavy, move the bag onto the floor or a nearby table. If you need help, ask for it.
8. Imagine that a huge canvas bag is on your lap.
9. Open it and take out a huge comb or brush.
10. Comb your hair, then put the comb back into the bag.
11. Put this bag on the floor

Adaptation

1. For small movements, imagine a tiny bag with tiny objects.

NB It is usually helpful to do some work with participants' own bags, especially handbags, as people often like to keep them close and may resent early instructions to put them away from them.

WARM-UPS AND STARTERS

GETTING TO KNOW EACH OTHER 1

Focus Names and noticing each other; discussing interests

Time 10 minutes

Equipment Selection of postcards (more than one per person), representing hobbies and interests of people in the group (as per assessment forms); large table for group members to sit around

Activity

1. Names are stated around the group.
2. Group members select a postcard which represents a hobby or interest.
3. They find other people who have similar interests or one they are interested in.
4. Discuss in pairs or small groups.
5. Round the group, members state names and interests.

Adaptation

1. Have a wider selection of postcards. People can also choose a postcard which shows some things they are not at all interested in. (This information may be useful when choosing later activities.)

WARM-UPS AND STARTERS

GETTING TO KNOW EACH OTHER 2

Focus Disclosing information about self; getting to know each other

Time 10 minutes

Equipment A large cardboard box, pens and papers

Activity

1 Pen and paper are given to each person.

2 Write on separate sheets of paper
(a) the most exciting thing I have done,
(b) the most wonderful day of my life,
(c) the biggest surprise I have ever had,
(d) my favourite food.

3 Fold up the pieces of paper, and put them into the box.

4 Take out the pieces of paper, one by one, and guess who wrote the item.

Adaptations

1 Staying with positives only, select other 'mosts'.

2 Draw instead of writing.

WARM-UPS AND STARTERS

GETTING TO KNOW EACH OTHER 3

Focus Getting to know others; hand flexibility

Time 10 minutes

Equipment List of star signs and their elements, sheets of paper, felt-tip pens, a large table for people to sit around

Activity

1. Each person writes their name at the top of their paper
2. Under this they draw their zodiac sign. (You may need to give this information to some people, who may be unaware of the symbol.)
3. Decide which are the fire, air, water and earth signs.
4. Divide participants into fire, air, water and earth signs.
5. Each group decides the good and helpful aspects of their element.
6. Each group creates a short hand mime to show their element.
7. Groups show these mimes to each other and state the positive aspects they have thought of.

Adaptations

1. Create an elements debate about the usefulness of each one.
2. Decide on the way the elements complement each other.

WARM-UPS AND STARTERS

GETTING TO KNOW EACH OTHER 4

Focus Names

Time 10 minutes

Equipment Pens and card, large table for people to sit around

Activity

1. Each person writes their name on a card. This should be the name they want to be called by in the group.
2. Each person places the card in front of them.
3. Each person says their name, repeating it twice.
4. Place the cards, blank side uppermost, together in the centre of the table and shuffle them.
5. Each person takes a card. (If people select their own, they should replace it and then choose another.)
6. Group members negotiate placing cards in front of the correct people. Individuals should not actively look for their own name; it is more helpful to become engaged in finding the owners of other names.
7. When everyone has their own name back in front of them, repeat the names.

WARM-UPS AND STARTERS

GETTING TO KNOW EACH OTHER 5

Focus Names, co-operation

Time 10 minutes

Equipment Felt-tip pens, large sheet of paper, large table for group members to sit around

Activity

1. Write your name on the paper. (Encourage people to write anywhere on the paper, not just on the edge nearest to them.)
2. Draw a flower shape around your name.
3. Look at the other flowers on the paper.
4. With everyone drawing, create a large group picture of a garden.
5. Each person points out their original flower, states their name and says how their flower fits in with the rest of the garden flowers and other items drawn.

Adaptations

1. Have paper on the floor and use brushes and paints (see page 12).
2. Discuss the atmosphere in the garden and talk about how it may feel to walk around in it.

WARM-UPS AND STARTERS

GETTING TO KNOW EACH OTHER 6

Focus Getting to know each other, finger dexterity

Time 10 minutes

Equipment String or nytrim, large table to sit around

Activity

1. Each person states their name.
2. Give each person a 12-inch length of string or nytrim.
3. Each person puts the nytrim or string into the shape of the first letter of their name.
4. Group members arrange these in alphabetical order in the centre of the table. This involves negotiation for each initial's place.
5. Members undo their shape and form the string into the first letter of their birthplace. They declaire the place to the group, adding their name.
6. They undo these shapes in turn and make a pleasing shape.
7. Put the shapes together in the centre of the table to form a group shape.

Adaptations

1. Add music to making shapes. Allow shapes to be influenced by different types of music.
2. Make a group shape on a large fabric sheet. Stick the shapes to the sheet and hang it on the wall for group sessions.
3. Make a maze from shapes and use fingers to 'walk' around the maze.

WARM-UPS AND STARTERS

GETTING TO KNOW EACH OTHER 7

Focus Names, noticing other people

Time 15 minutes

Equipment Envelopes, pre-written (enough for each group member to have one for every other member), paper, pens

Activity

1. Members state their names.
2. Each person notices something they like about other group members. It may be an item of clothing, their voice, their smile — anything they like.
3. Write a short note to each person, saying what it is that you like about them.
4. Put the notes in the correct envelopes.
5. Select some group members to be letter deliverers.
6. They deliver the letters.
7. When they have all been delivered, everyone opens their letters and reads them out.

Adaptations

1. Group members address envelopes.
2. Instead of letters, make illustrated cards with a note inside.

WARM-UPS AND STARTERS

GETTING TO KNOW EACH OTHER 8

Focus Expertise of people in the group, names

Time 15 minutes

Equipment Large sheet of paper, felt-tip pens

Activity

1. Draw a road which goes from one side of the paper to the other. (This may be done with each person drawing a section, then joining them.)
2. As a group, decide what kind of traveller might be travelling on this road. Draw the traveller.
3. Consider the difficulties that the traveller might meet on the journey.
4. Each participant comes up with one difficulty. (This should be a difficulty that the person has knowledge of.)
5. Offer advice to the traveller.

Adaptations

1. Make a puppet traveller and manipulate the puppet to travel the road and stop and ask advice.
2. Decide on the quest that the traveller is undertaking and offer suggestions on how to reach the destination.

WARM-UPS AND STARTERS

GETTING TO KNOW EACH OTHER 9

Focus Creativity, learning more about other group members

Time 15 minutes

Equipment Large sheet of paper, table for people to sit around

Activity

1. Individuals state their names to the group.
2. On the large sheet of paper, draw a very large circle. Divide it into four. Mark each quarter with a different season.
3. Group members decide on their favourite season.
4. Draw items from these seasons in the appropriate quarters of the circle.
5. Each group introduces their season and talks about the kinds of things they do or used to do during these seasons.

Adaptations

1. Break down seasons into festivals and special events.
2. Mime some of the events people describe.

WARM-UPS AND STARTERS

GETTING TO KNOW EACH OTHER 10

Focus Knowing other people's tastes; collaboration

Time 15 minutes

Equipment Large table for people to sit around, card and felt-tip pens

Activity

1. Each person writes their name at the top of their card.
2. In turn round the groups, individuals call out their names.
3. Each person writes four of their favourite food items on the cards (*not* complete dishes, such as stew, fish and chips or casserole, but food items such as beef, fish, jelly or peas).
4. They read these out.
5. The group creates a three or four course meal that will incorporate these. Other items can be added.

Adaptations

1. Create a banquet for a special occasion.
2. Creat different kinds of menus for other groups: children, old people and so on.

WARM-UPS AND STARTERS

THE ENVIRONMENT 1

Focus Becoming familiar with the room; imaginative processes

Time 10 minutes

Equipment None

Activity

1. Notice the arrangement of chairs, tables and other furniture. Decide on the effect of the colours in the room.
2. Imagine the room having different functions:
   (a) a doctor's waiting room,
   (b) a hotel reception area,
   (c) a magnificent room in a mansion.
3. Group members suggest another room.
4. Divide into pairs or small groups and decide how the furniture would be different. What colours would be changed?
5. Pairs/small groups feed back into the group.

Adaptations

1. Draw a room map and then draw a second map showing the change in the room function.
2. Suggest the types of people who could be in the imagined rooms.

WARM-UPS AND STARTERS

THE ENVIRONMENT 2

Focus Getting to know the room and the route to it

Time 15 minutes

Equipment Felt-tip pens and paper

Activity

1. Members describe the room or place they were in before the group.
2. They describe their journey to the room.
3. Each person draws a map of their journey to the room.
4. They describe to the group, or one or two other people, who they met on the way. Did they notice anything else during the journey?
5. As a group, create a map that shows all the journeys.

Adaptations

1. Add mimes of one of the activities they were engaged in before the group.
2. Add the journey they will be making after the group.

WARM-UPS AND STARTERS

THE ENVIRONMENT 3

Focus Becoming familiar with the room, finding space in the room

Time 15 minutes

Equipment None

Activity

1. Look around the room and notice inviting places.
2. Identify which places are the best source of light, comfort and interest.
3. Move to the selected area.
4. Stay in this area for a while and think about why it is nice to be there.
5. Return to the group and report back. How can group placings incorporate some of these areas?

Adaptations

1. Add unpleasant areas. Sit in them. How can we avoid these areas during group time?
2. Half of the group sit in their comfortable area and invite members from the other half to visit them in this place. Reverse the procedure.

WARM-UPS AND STARTERS

THE ENVIRONMENT 4

Focus Knowing the room, movement through it

Time 15 minutes

Equipment Felt-tip pens and paper

Activity

1. Draw an outline of the room, adding furniture.
2. Group members decide on any reasons for leaving the room that may occur during group time. (This may include visits to the toilet or collecting something that has been forgotten.)
3. Discuss what reasons for leaving may be permissible in this group. How can we avoid forgetting things?
4. When permissible reasons have been identified, draw routes for reaching the required destination on the plan:
   (a) quickest, safest route,
   (b) most difficult route,
   (c) most interesting route.
5. Try out the routes.
6. Return to the group.

Adaptations

1. Use string or nytrim on the floor to show the routes.
2. Make a large, colourful map to show the routes. Keep it on the wall for future groups.

WARM-UPS AND STARTERS

THE ENVIRONMENT 5

Focus Becoming familiar with the room; discussion and imagination

Time 10 minutes

Equipment None

Activity

1. Look or walk slowly around the room.
2. Notice blank spaces on the walls.
3. Choose one space that interests you: it can be small or large.
4. Think about a painting that you would like to see there. It may be one you know or from your imagination.
5. Share your ideas with others. Say why it would look nice on the wall.

Adaptations

1. Group leaders have postcards of paintings; they ask the group to decide where they would hang the actual painting, and why.
2. Add other ideas for wall decoration: mirrors, plants and so on. Where would people like them?

WARM-UPS AND STARTERS

THE ENVIRONMENT 6

Focus Getting to know the room; observation

Time 10 minutes

Equipment Felt-tip pens and paper

Activity

1. Notice the furniture in the room. Discuss it with a partner.
2. Close your eyes or look down.
3. Group leaders change three things about the room (for example, they move chairs, remove a picture and remove the table covering).
4. Open your eyes and write the changes on your paper.
5. Discuss.

Adaptations

1. Group members take it in turns to change items in the room or to suggest changes for leaders to make. Other group members keep their eyes closed while the changes are made and then have to spot what they were.
2. Instead of changing furniture around, add three items while members have their eyes closed. Ask group members to discover the added items.

WARM-UPS AND STARTERS

THE ENVIRONMENT 7

Focus Becoming familiar with the room; developing imagination

Time 15 minutes

Equipment Felt-tip pens and paper

Activity

1. Notice all of the doors and windows in the room.
2. Write adjectives that describe them. Are they wooden, colourful, large, small?
3. What is on the other side of each window and door? Ask other people to look and report if you are unsure.
4. Choose one door or window.
5. Imagine that this leads to a beautiful garden. Draw the garden. (This can be done by an individual, in pairs or in groups.)
6. Describe the garden to others.
7. Return to the window or door to confirm what is actually there.

Adaptations

1. Draw four pictures of the garden, one for each season.
2. Talk about actual gardens that people know.
3. Have postcards of gardens available, and discuss or draw how these might look in different seasons.

NB Be wary of this kind of exercise with people who are confused. It may be more helpful for them to draw what is actually beyond the door or window.

WARM-UPS AND STARTERS

THE ENVIRONMENT 8

Focus Becoming familiar with the environment; developing imagination

Time 15 minutes

Equipment Felt-tip pens and paper

Activity

1. Divide into groups of four or five people, with *at least one* ambulant person per group.
2. Each group draws an outline of the room and adds furniture and fittings to the room plan.
3. One 'runner' per group is chosen and is sent to different room areas to check details.
4. Two colours are chosen: one for safety and one for danger. The 'runner' is sent to confirm areas of safety and danger which are then added to the plan.
5. Groups report back.

Adaptations

1. Add sound to the report on areas of safety and danger.
2. Creat a fictional character to make a journey around the room at different times of day and night. Recount the journey. Do areas of safety and danger change according to the time?

WARM-UPS AND STARTERS

THE ENVIRONMENT 9

Focus Becoming familiar with the environment; developing imagination

Time 10 minutes

Equipment None

Activity

1. Look around the room. Notice surfaces that a vase could be placed on.
2. Each person imagines the most beautiful bouquet of flowers.
3. When everyone is ready, each person describes the flowers in their bouquet.
4. What kind of vase would you put the bouquet in?
5. Whereabouts in this room would you place the vase of flowers and why? How would it change the room? What effect would the colours have?

Adaptations

1. With coloured pens and paper, draw the flowers and vase.
2. Mime the shape of the vase.

WARM-UPS AND STARTERS

THE ENVIRONMENT 10

Focus Becoming familiar with the room; developing imagination

Time 10 minutes

Equipment None

Activity

1. Look around the room.
2. Imagine that the room is to be cleared to create a huge space in the middle.
3. Decide which items will be the heaviest to lift, which will be the most bulky, the most difficult to lift, the most awkward and so on.
4. Decide on the order of moving the furniture. How would items fit together round the edge of the room? Which spaces should not be blocked?
5. Imagine the floor space is now clear. What could happen in this large space? (Dances, games and so on.)
6. Mime some of these activities from chairs or from a standing position.

Adaptations

1. How could fragile items be packed?
2. Make maps of full and cleared areas.

MOVING INTO DRAMA

STORYMAKING 1

Focus Dramatic imagination; overcoming obstacles; communication

Time 30–35 minutes

Equipment Selection of postcards, people, heroes, heroines, villains, landscapes

Activity

1. Divide into small groups of three or four.
2. Each group chooses a postcard that represents an ideal landscape or a beautiful place.
3. Each group places this postcard on the table, leaving a large space between themselves and the postcard.
4. Each group now chooses a postcard that shows a figure for their hero or heroine.
5. This postcard is placed on the table near to the group.
6. Each group chooses two postcards of figures who are villains.
7. Place these between the landscape and the hero/heroine.
8. Decide on the reason the hero/heroine has for making a journey to the ideal landscape. Decide on the hero's/heroine's name and their qualities. Which qualities will enable them to complete the journey?
9. Decide on the reasons the villains have for obstructing the hero's/heroine's journey.
10. Create the story of the hero's/heroine's journey to the ideal land. How do they overcome the obstructions that the villains present? What does the hero/heroine do when they reach the ideal land?
11. Share the stories.

Adaptation

1. Dramatize some aspects of the story, such as the meeting with the villains, the preparation for the journey and arriving in the beautiful land.

MOVING INTO DRAMA

STORYMAKING 2

Focus Hand/arm co-ordination, imagination, co-operation, concentration

Time 30–40 minutes

Equipment Large sticks

Activity

1. Warm up, in a seated position, by handling sticks and putting them into different positions as suggested by the group leader.
2. Divide into small groups of three or four people.
3. In small groups, place the sticks in different positions.
4. Create three shapes with the sticks, which are to be touching in some way.
5. Recreate these three shapes twice.
6. Create a story around these three shapes.
7. Share the story with other groups, creating the stick shapes as they are mentioned in the story.

Adaptations

1. Use small objects such as straws or plastic spoons.
2. Create a central character to build the story around.

MOVING INTO DRAMA

STORYMAKING 3

Focus Co-operation, communication, imagination

Time 30–35 minutes

Equipment Postcards of doors and gates, felt-tip pens, paper, large table

Activity

1. Group members look at postcards.
2. Divide into small groups of three or four people.
3. Each group selects one card depicting a gate and one of a door.
4. Each group decides what lies behind the door and then imagines the gate as the gate to the garden that surrounds the building which the door belongs to.
5. Draw the building and the garden.
6. Give the group members the start of the story: 'One day a traveller arrived at your building...'
7. Each group decides on its traveller.
8. The next stage of the story: 'The traveller is seeking a treasure in the building but must first overcome a trap set for them in the garden.'
9. The groups decide on their treasure and trap.
10. They create the story of how the traveller finds the treasure and what is done with it.
11. Share the stories.

MOVING INTO DRAMA

STORYMAKING 4

Focus Co-ordination, co-operation; imaginative process; perception

Time 30–35 minutes

Equipment Lengths of nytrim, large sheets of paper, paints, brushes and a large table

Activity

1. Each group member makes a shape from a length of nytrim.
2. Group members look at each shape and make suggestions about what they could be: for example, a round shape could be a pool of water, a mirror, a ring or a ship's porthole.
3. Spread large sheets of paper onto the floor or table.
4. Group members take longer pieces of nytrim and throw them onto the sheets of paper.
5. What do the shapes that the nytrim makes remind people of?
6. Use the paints to complete the picture.
7. Divide into small groups and focus on the created objects.
8. Create a story around these objects.
9. Each small group shares their story with the others.
10. Reflect on the stories.

Adaptations

1. Give one of the objects magical properties.
2. Add sounds, such as that of a bee around a flower or the rippling of a pool when the wind blows. Add sounds to the story when it is being told.

MOVING INTO DRAMA

STORYMAKING 5

Focus Co-operation; tactile sensations; finger and hand flexibility

Time 30–35 minutes

Equipment A selection of large fabric pieces, a large table

Activity

1. Have the fabric pieces on the table. Invite group members to touch the fabric and hold them to different parts of their body to feel the different sensations and textures.
2. Hold fabrics in different positions to add shadow and light. Notice how the surface or sheen changes.
3. Place the fabric in shapes that reflect the shadows and the light.
4. Look at the shapes. What kind of landscape do the combined shapes suggest?
5. Decide on the kinds of things that people might do in this terrain.
6. In small groups, decide on a story that takes place in this terrain.
7. Tell these stories.
8. Reflect on the stories.

Adaptations

1. Have a range of small plastic animals for people to place in the landscape. Tell the story of the animals.
2. Show how the landscape looks in different seasons.

MOVING INTO DRAMA

STORYMAKING 6

Focus Co-operation, perception, imagination

Time 30–35 minutes

Equipment Postcards showing groups of four or five people, a large table

Activity

1. Allow group members time to look at the postcards.
2. Divide into small groups. Each group selects one postcard.
3. Each group resolves the following questions: Who are the people? What are they doing? Where are they? Why are they there? When is this scene taking place (year, season, day, time of day)?
4. Create the story of the events that happened before and after the scene shown on the postcard.
5. Share the postcards and stories with other groups.
6. Reflect on the stories.

Adaptations

1. Choose the postcard selection so that each group of people shown includes some seated people. Groups take up the postures of the people shown on the card and tell the story as the postcard characters.
2. Tell the story from the different points of view of the people in the postcard.

MOVING INTO DRAMA

STORYMAKING 7

Focus Co-operation; imagination; views of age and gender

Time 30–35 minutes

Equipment None

Activity

1. Provide the following story outline. The scene is a cobbled street, flanked on either side by tall, four-storey houses. Walking down the street is a young woman, carrying a large parcel; she is dressed in beautiful clothes. She is followed by a very old man, who carries a large folder. He is dressed in black. Following them is an old woman, covered in a huge cloak, accompanied by a young man who carries a huge bag. They do not speak to each other. Each person walks with a sure step as if they are on the point of arriving at their destinations.
2. In small groups decide who the characters are and what are their relationships to each other.
3. Decide on their destinations and what the items they carry contain.
4. Create the story of their journeys.
5. Share the stories with other group members.
6. Reflect on the stories.

Adaptations

1. Give the information that one character is not an ordinary human being but has magical powers: which character and what magical powers?
2. Group members create a tableau of the characters; each tells the story as the character they represent.
3. Provide information about the destination and an obstacle to prevent them reaching it. How do they overcome the obstacle?

MOVING INTO DRAMA

STORYMAKING 8

Focus Perception, concentration, imagination; co-operation

Time 30–40 minutes

Equipment A large key, a mirror, a glove, a book, pens and paper

Activity

1. Have the objects arranged on a table.
2. In pairs, or as individuals, write down adjectives for each item.
3. Divide into small groups and decide upon a place where all of these items can be found.
4. Create two characters who might own these objects.
5. It is a special day for one of the characters. What is that day?
6. Why are these objects together for this day?
7. Prepare the story of the day, including all the objects.
8. Share the stories.
9. Reflect on the stories.

Adaptations

1. Create particular forms of stories from the objects: a murder mystery, a ghost story, a romance, and so on.
2. Make one of the objects a magical item, and create a story that reveals its magic.
3. Vary the collection of items to create different kinds of story.

MOVING INTO DRAMA

STORYMAKING 9

Focus Perception, reworking familiar concepts, concern

Time 30–35 minutes

Equipment Large sheets of paper, pens

Activity

1. Using paper and pens, brainstorm the titles of folk or fairy stories.
2. Recall the plots of some of these stories.
3. Recount the ending to these tales in detail.
4. Decide on the most popular tale.
5. Divide into small groups and devise different endings. (For example, the slipper in *Cinderella* fits one of the ugly sisters, or perhaps Cinderella decides she does not want to marry the prince. What happens next?)
6. Tell the revised stories to other group members.

MOVING INTO DRAMA

STORYMAKING 10

Focus Co-operation, co-ordination; arm, finger and hand co-ordination

Time 30–35 minutes

Equipment Instruments, jars and tins filled with small items to provide different sounds

Activity

1. Encourage group members to provide different kinds of sounds from the items provided.
2. In pairs or threes, create rhythms with the sounds.
3. Start to change the rhythms to the rhythms of footsteps: of a young child, of a man in a hurry, of a woman carrying heavy shopping. (The aim is to create the rhythm of these rather than to try to reproduce an exact sound.)
4. Experiment with creating other footstep rhythms.
5. Decide on four particular rhythms.
6. Create the personal details of the characters and decide what they are doing.
7. Create a story around the sounds and characters.
8. Share with others in the group the combination of sounds and story.
9. Reflect on the stories.

Adaptations

1. Add other sounds to the story action, for example a door closing.
2. Tell the story entirely with sounds.

MOVING INTO DRAMA

STORYMAKING 11

Focus Upper trunk, hand, arm and finger flexibility; imagination; co-ordination

Time 30–40 minutes

Equipment Instruments, jars of different items to provide a range of sounds, a large table

Activity

1. Have the sound-making items on the table. Encourage the group to experiment with them to produce sounds.
2. The group clap the beat of some songs known to them.
3. Half of the group clap the song beat while the other half create the beat with instruments. Reverse roles.
4. Think of some songs that tell a story.
5. Divide into small groups. Each group decides on their own song.
6. Decide who are the people in the song, including the person who is singing. (For example, who is the person singing to Daisy in 'Daisy, Daisy'?)
7. Create the story of what had happened before the song and what happened afterwards.
8. Practise creating the tune with the instruments (and singing if people know all the words).
9. Present the song and the story to other group members.
10. Reflect on the stories.

MOVING INTO DRAMA

STORYMAKING 12

Focus Co-ordination, co-operation, imagination and perception

Time 30–40 minutes

Equipment Felt-tip pens, paper, items to draw around for different shapes

Activity

1. Draw around various items to create a variety of shapes.
2. Move the paper into different positions to see shapes from different perspectives.
3. Move your hands around the shapes to frame them. How could we hold some of these shapes? In the palm of the hand? With two fingers? (And so on.)
4. Place your hands in different positions as if to hold different shapes.
5. Place your hands on blank sheets of paper and make different shapes with your hands.
6. Decide on one particular shape; with your free hand draw around this hand shape or keep your hand still for someone else to draw around it.
7. Look at these drawn hand shapes from different perspectives. What could these hands be holding or doing?
8. Divide into small groups and create stories around these hand shapes.
9. Tell the stories.
10. Reflect on the stories.

MOVING INTO DRAMA

STORYMAKING 13

Focus Co-ordination, communication; imagination and concentration

Time 30–40 minutes

Equipment Shoes, slippers, felt-tip pens, paper and a large table

Activity

1. Have the footwear on the table for people to handle. Feel the different materials and discuss functions of shoes: walking shoes, dancing shoes, and so on.
2. Group members place a shoe on a blank sheet of paper and draw around it to produce an outline on the paper.
3. They then colour in the outline.
4. Divide into small groups.
5. Each group imagines the type of person who might wear this shoe and devises a story about a journey that that person might undertake.
6. Tell the stories.
7. Reflect on the stories.

Adaptations

1. Create magic shoes that will fly, run, jump and take their owners into different worlds. Tell stories incorporating the above.
2. Put the shoes onto a magic carpet that journeys to fantastic lands.

MOVING INTO DRAMA

STORYMAKING 14

Focus Concentration, perception; imagination and communication

Time 30–35 minutes

Equipment Felt-tip pens and paper, clocks, if readily available

Activity

1. Look at the clocks or draw clocks and brainstorm different types.
2. Brainstorm sayings and proverbs about time.
3. Divide into small groups and create a magical clock.
4. Decide on the magic of the clock.
5. Create a story about the magical clock. When the hands stop, time stands still. For how long? How does this affect a character or characters?
6. Tell the stories.

Adaptations

1. Take other everyday objects and create a magical story from the function of the object.
2. Use a grandmother or grandfather clock as the magic item. The clock has a door to another world. What happens when a person enters the clock?

MOVING INTO DRAMA

STORYMAKING 15

Focus Communication, imagination and concentration

Time 30–35 minutes

Equipment Pens and paper, a large table

Activity

1. Brainstorm proverbs and sayings.
2. Divide into small groups and choose people's favourite proverbs or sayings.
3. Create stories to illustrate each member's choice.
4. Share the stories.
5. Reflect on the sayings.

Adaptations

1. Tell stories for other group members to guess the proverb the story illustrates.

Through participating in these storymaking activities (pages 87–101), groups usually create beautiful, imaginative stories and may want these to be shared with others outside the group. There are various possibilities:

(a) Type the stories and illustrate them; keep them in a folder or in book form.
(b) Create special stories for children known to people in the group. Make some of the stories into posters for group members to give to the children.
(c) Hold a story-telling afternoon or evening. Group members can tell the stories to an invited audience (very useful if the group will be moving on to performance work).
(d) Make stories into posters to hang on the wall.
(e) Employ an artist to illustrate some of the stories for use as wall hangings or pictures.

MOVING INTO DRAMA

DRAMATIC SCENARIOS 1

Focus Movement; creative imagination; co-operation, communication

Time 30–35 minutes

Equipment A collection of hats, large table

Conditions Physical warm-up

Activity

1. Have the hats arranged on the table.
2. Encourage participants to look at hats and try them on.
3. As people try on the hats, they take on the posture of the person who might wear this hat. For example, a person wearing a top hat will probably be standing straight and be dignified; a beret might represent a schoolgirl walking slowly to school or hurrying away.
4. Divide the hats into those that people who might be seated would wear and hats that suggest activity.
5. Participants choose appropriate hats. Those wearing hats representing activity move around the room; other participants remain seated. Everyone allows their hat to dictate their movement and activity.
6. Participants who are moving start to interact with those seated, acting as the characters suggested by the hats.
7. Divide into small groups, comprised of active and sedentary participants.
8. Share information about characters within the small group.
9. Decide why the characters are together, where they are, when their meeting is taking place and what might happen during their meeting.
10. Create a short scene about these characters.
11. Share these scenes with other group members.
12. Replace the hats on the table and leave the aspects of the assumed character with them.
13. Reflect on the drama.

MOVING INTO DRAMA

DRAMATIC SCENARIOS 2

Focus Co-ordination, flexibility; concentration, communication, dramatic imagination

Time 30–35 minutes

Equipment Music with varying rhythms

Conditions Hands and arms warm-up

Activity

1. Move hands and wrists to slow, soft music (the leader may need to lead the movement).
2. Extend the movement to include arms and shoulders.
3. Rest your arms and hands. Move your feet to the music.
4. With a change of music to a marching rhythm, move your feet and legs to the beat.
5. In small groups make arm and hand movements to the marching rhythm. Start to interact with others via the movement. (The leader stops the music.)
6. Imagine that in the centre of each group there are two huge mixing bowls and a tin. A very special cake is to be baked.
7. Each small group decides on the special occasion.
8. Mime rolling up sleeves and putting on aprons.
9. Continue miming:
   - (a) Grease and line a very large baking tin. Put it to one side.
   - (b) Put raisins, sultanas, currants, peel, almonds and cherries into the first bowl. Finger movements show the different shapes of the fruit.
   - (c) Into the other bowl sift flour, spices and salt; mix well together.
   - (d) Cream butter and then add sugar and beat.
   - (e) Break eggs on the side of the bowl.
   - (f) Fold the eggs into the mixture.
   - (g) Fold the dry ingredients into the mixture.
   - (h) Add any other special ingredient, such as brandy or extra spices.
   - (i) Turn the mixture into the prepared tin.
   - (j) Put the tin into the oven.
   - (k) Wash your hands.

MOVING INTO DRAMA

DRAMATIC SCENARIOS 2 (*Continued*)

Activity

10 Decide on a decoration for the cake.

11 Continue the mime: remove the cake from the oven and put it into a very special, super-fast cooling machine.

12 Prepare the icing and other decorations.

13 Take the cake from the cooling machine and decorate it.

14 Decide how the cake is to be displayed for the occasion.

15 Each group describes their completed cake and the display area to the others.

16 They reflect on special cakes that they have baked or had baked for them.

17 Close with a group description of a cake they would like to bake and decorate for this group.

MOVING INTO DRAMA

DRAMATIC SCENARIOS 3

Focus Movement and speech patterns; co-operation, communication; making choices

Time 30 minutes

Equipment Large sheet of paper, pens

Activity

1. On the large sheet of paper, the whole group write as many colours as they can think of. Leave large spaces between the colours.
2. When the group have completed this, they write connections with the colours near to the word, such as red—energy, danger; blue—cool, comforting and so on.
3. Each group member chooses a colour.
4. Divide into small groups.
5. Each person shares information about their chosen colour and the words connected with it.
6. Each person creates a character from the chosen colour; for example, a person who chose red may be an energetic, dangerous person, or other words the group has chosen for red may apply.
7. People talk about their characters.
8. Find a posture and movement for the characters.
9. Talk about the weather, in general terms, as the characters allow the colour adjectives to influence their voices. For example, does the character speak quickly, loudly, softly or in a murmur?
10. The group leader tells participants that they are all in a waiting area. They have been called together to receive a huge surprise. The news has come from 'a well-wisher'. They do not know what the surprise is. The waiting area is very comfortable.

MOVING INTO DRAMA

DRAMATIC SCENARIOS 3 (*Continued*)

Activity

11 In the small groups, as the chosen characters, participants discuss their reactions to the news and talk about their journeys to the waiting area.

12 Characters discuss what they hope for as a surprise.

13 The group leader announces that the surprise is a million pounds for each participant, to be given to a charity of their choice.

14 Discuss the charities that the money is to be given to and why.

15 Group members de-role by resuming their own posture and own speech patterns.

16 The large group discusses the charities that the money was given to and how the characters came to their decision.

MOVING INTO DRAMA

DRAMATIC SCENARIOS 4

Focus Co-operation, movement, dramatic imagination

Time 30–35 minutes

Equipment Large table, large sheet of paper, pens, sound-making items

Activity

1. Have the large sheet of paper on the table. On one side group members draw the sun and, on the other, the moon.
2. Write words connected with the moon on the moon part of the paper and words connected with the sun on the other.
3. Divide into two groups: one to become moon characters, the other to become sun characters. There is one leader per group.
4. Focus on the words on the paper and move into postures which represent these words.
5. Each group creates sounds from the instruments provided to represent the sun or the moon. Group leaders may need to lead with sounds for group members to add to.
6. Create movement and sound to represent the rising, shining and setting of the sun or moon.
7. Devise a sequence of sound and movement which depicts the simultaneous setting of the sun and rising of the moon, and the setting of the moon and the rising of the sun.
8. The two groups work together to depict dusk and dawn.
9. Repeat with increased sound and movement.
10. Reflect on the action.

MOVING INTO DRAMA

DRAMATIC SCENARIOS 5

Focus Co-ordination, co-operation, communication; movement, recognition

Time 30–35 minutes

Equipment Nytrim: one long piece, also one shorter length for each group member

Activity

1 Place nytrim on the floor, arranged as a circle. The group sit round the circle.

2 Imagine the circle as an island. What shape would the group like this island to be? Change the shape of the nytrim until everyone is satisfied.

3 Give each group member a short length of nytrim.

4 Members make the short lengths of nytrim into things that might be on the island, such as trees, swamps and temples, and place them in the island shape or instruct someone else to place them in position.

5 They view the complete structure from different positions around the shape.

6 Divide into small groups and move into different parts of the room.

7 Each group is a group of travellers in a boat sailing towards the island. Arrange the chairs to form the boats.

8 Decide who the people in the boat are and why they are sailing to the island. For example, they are a group of shipwrecked people sailing towards safety, or a group of pirates looking for treasure.

9 Assume the postures of the characters in the boats.

10 Create conversation between the characters about the island they are sailing towards.

11 Wait until communication between the characters has been established. The people in the boats see the island and decide upon an advance party.

12 The different advance parties reach the island and explore.

MOVING INTO DRAMA

DRAMATIC SCENARIOS 5 (*Continued*)

Activity

13 The characters in the boats call out questions to their advance party and they are answered.

14 The groups negotiate with each other via the advance parties regarding the part of the island they will settle on.

15 The advance parties return to the boats and report their findings.

16 In small groups, the characters discuss how they will settle on the island and how they will survive.

17 Elect a spokesperson from each group.

18 The spokespeople travel back to the island and negotiate their settlement.

19 They report back to the characters in the group.

20 De-role and return to the large group.

21 In the large group, reflect on the drama.

Adaptation

1 Add the concept of a year passing and devise the story of how the groups lived together on the island.

MOVING INTO DRAMA

DRAMATIC SCENARIOS 6

Focus Co-ordination, co-operation, communication; movement, recognition

Time 30–35 minutes

Equipment Lengths of nytrim

Activity

1. Place a long length of nytrim on the floor to make a maze shape.
2. Think about and discuss mazes in stories and mazes that exist in fact and myth.
3. Divide into small groups, each of which creates a maze of nytrim.
4. Decide on the treasure that is hidden in the centre of the maze.
5. Decide on the place where the maze is sited and why it was created.
6. Decide who are the treasure seekers and why they are seeking the treasure.
7. How do they prepare to enter the maze? In order to enter, they must create a rhythm to move to, first with hands clapping, then with feet.
8. Moving to this rhythm the travellers enter the maze.
9. The seekers find the treasure in the centre of the maze. It can only be removed by the creation of a different rhythm.
10. The treasure seekers create the next rhythm and move the treasure.
11. Outside the maze, they open the treasure box and examine the contents with exclamations of delight.
12. The seekers decide what to do with the treasure.
13. De-role by moving the nytrim.
14. Reflect on the drama.

MOVING INTO DRAMA

DRAMATIC SCENARIOS 7

Focus Movement, expressing emotion

Time 30–35 minutes

Equipment None

Conditions Physical warm-up

Activity

1. The group are sitting or standing with space around each individual.
2. Ask group members to assume the shape of:
   (a) a person who has received good news,
   (b) a person who has received bad news,
   (c) a person who is anxious about some exam results,
   (d) a person who is very tired,
   (e) a person who is about to express extreme anger.
   Relax between each shape.
3. In groups of three or four, make the shape of a statue representing great joy.
4. Change the shape to that of the group's conception of 'a great escape'. Relax.
5. Move the shape to express freedom. Relax.
6. Still in the small groups, decide the kind of place people could be trapped in.
7. Create the shape of the trapped people.
8. Improvise the kinds of things they could be saying.
9. Move into the escape shape. Improvise the things people escaping may be saying.
10. Move into the freedom shape. Add sounds and words to the shape.
11. Share these dramas with other group members.
12. Reflect on the dramas and the feelings of being trapped, escaping and freedom.

MOVING INTO DRAMA

DRAMATIC SCENARIOS 8

Focus Exploration of relationship between different age groups; advice giving

Time 30–35 minutes

Equipment Large and small sheets of paper, pens, table

Conditions Physical warm-up

Activity

1. Brainstorm sayings and proverbs that provide advice.
2. On small sheets of paper, each person writes one number between 10 and 25 and one between 50 and 80. Fold these and place them on the table.
3. Divide into pairs.
4. Each pair takes one piece of folded paper. The two numbers represent the ages of the pair.
5. Sitting or standing, they assume postures that show the characters' age.
6. Decide on the relationship between the two people, and who will be the advice giver.
7. The advice giver gives advice in the form of sayings and proverbs. The other person reflects the advice. After a short interaction the advice giver moves onto the next piece of advice. This is also reflected. Continue.
8. Reverse roles.
9. Pairs, as themselves, select a proverb that they feel offers useful advice.
10. Feed back these proverbs into the large group.
11. Reflect on the drama.

MOVING INTO DRAMA

DRAMATIC SCENARIOS 9

Focus Movement; communication of abstract thought; changing perceptions

Time 30–35 minutes

Equipment Collection of hats, large table, coloured pens and paper

Conditions Physical warm-up

Activity

1. Have the hats displayed on the table.
2. Encourage group members to look at and touch the hats.
3. Try on the hats and notice how they feel.
4. Replace the hats on the table.
5. With pens and a large sheet of paper, brainstorm characters that people connect with hats, such as the Mad Hatter, Sherlock Holmes, court jesters and dons.
6. Decide how hats can suggest or define the status of the wearer.
7. Draw some fantastic hats on sheets of paper.
8. Decide on a magical property for each drawn hat.
9. Divide into small groups. They create some ordinary characters and decide where they are. What are they doing? Where do they find the magic hats?
10. Each group creates a short scene:
    (a) The ordinary characters are going about their everyday tasks.
    (b) They interact with each other in a friendly, talkative way.
    (c) They find the hats.
    (d) How do they react to the hats?
    (e) What kind of actions do they use to place the hats on their heads?
    (f) How does the magic happen?
    (g) What happens next?
    (h) People remove the hats and return to their everyday tasks.
    (i) The characters rest and talk about their experiences with the magic hats.
11. Members de-role by making their own everyday movements, yawn and stretch.
12. In the large group, reflect on the drama.

MOVING INTO DRAMA

DRAMATIC SCENARIOS 10

Focus Movement; expressing emotions, communication

Time 30–40 minutes

Equipment Song sheets

Activity

1. Group members focus on outings. What kind of outings do people go on?

2. Discuss groups of people who might go on an outing, such as a works outing, a club or society outing.

3. Decide on the outing group and destination for the group activity this session.

4. Which particular characters may be going on the outing, and what traits may they have? Examples might include an anxious organizer, a timid, travel-sick club/group secretary, a bossy driver.

5. Lay out chairs to form the interior of the coach.

6. The driver boards the coach, followed by the outing organizer. The other characters board the coach.

7. Everyone settles and anticipates arriving at their destination.

8. Group leaders call out the following instructions (avoid all instructions calling for sudden movement):
   - (a) The bus is difficult to get started: first attempt, everyone jolts forward; second attempt, bus shudders and everyone reacts; third attempt, bus moves hesitantly forward.
   - (b) Bus swerves suddenly to the right. Everyone reacts in slow motion.
   - (c) Bus goes over a road being repaired, *in slow motion*. People react to the bumpy road.
   - (d) A packed lunch is passed around. Passengers eat and drink, comment on the food.
   - (e) The driver realizes they are lost. The organizer tries to calm cross passengers.
   - (f) The organizer realizes that the maps have been left behind.
   - (g) The driver becomes cross, the passengers talk angrily among themselves.
   - (h) The organizer tries to calm everyone.

MOVING INTO DRAMA

DRAMATIC SCENARIOS 10 (*Continued*)

Activity

(i) The driver announces that the coach has run out of fuel.
(j) Some members get out to push the coach into a lay-by.
(k) As the volunteers push, others call out a pushing rhyme.
(l) During the wait for assistance there is a sing-song (leaders produce some song sheets).
(m) The driver remembers the reserve cans of fuel. The tank is filled.
(n) Cheers from the passengers.
(o) The driver announces that he or she is not prepared to continue the journey.
(p) The passengers argue but the driver remains adamant.
(q) The coach returns home, with disgruntled passengers.
(r) The passengers leave the coach with a very discontented air.

9 De-role by shaking arms and hands and moving chairs to dismantle the coach.

10 Reflect on the drama. Recall outings group members have been on.

MOVING INTO DRAMA

DRAMATIC SCENARIOS 11

Focus Flexibility; co-operation, co-ordination; concentration; exploring life cycles, ways of overcoming difficulties

Time 30–40 minutes

Equipment Postcards of trees, a large table

Conditions Physical warm-up

Activity

1. Have the postcards arranged on a table. Encourage participants to look at them.
2. Group members choose their favourite postcards.
3. Place these where everyone can see them, or pass them around the group.
4. Sitting or standing, group members take up tree postures. Encourage people to spread their arms as branches. Imagine that the roots grow deeply down into the ground.
5. The 'trees' start to react to the strong wind.
6. Resting in between each activity, take group members through the seasons.
   (a) Spring—buds appear, birds start to nest, roots become nourished and grow.
   (b) Summer—blossom and leaves abound. Bees buzz around for pollen. Reach out to the sun and receive the light summer showers with happiness. Feel the sap flowing through the trunk.
   (c) Autumn—leaves start to fall, birds begin to migrate, there is heavy rain and it is cold.
   (d) Winter—some trees have bare branches and some animals hibernate, needing protection from the trees.
   (e) Spring—leaves start to grow and the sun starts to shine again.
7. Divide into four small groups: one group per season. Think about the different kinds of trees. Use postcards that the group have chosen as an aid. People may not keep to the cycle used before: some trees keep their leaves all year round.
8. Each group member decides on their 'tree mood' during their chosen season.

DRAMATIC SCENARIOS 11 (*Continued*)

Activity

9 Decide on the place where the trees are living. Still in the small groups, create a vivid description of this place.

10 Group members 'become' the trees in this place. Pay attention to the spacial relationships of the trees: are they close together or apart? How does the chosen season affect their postures?

11 In roles as the trees, the group members discuss what they consider to be the greatest danger to them. What would most threaten their survivial?

12 Relax and consider how the trees might cope with dangers. How will the chosen season affect their responses and who might threaten their survival?

13 Rehearse a scene which follows this order:
(a) The trees are safe in their environment. By word and action, they show the season.
(b) The trees sense danger. Members show this in their bodies and a few words.
(c) The danger arrives. Show the trees' reactions. Call on help, if available.
(d) The danger is overcome.
(e) The trees are safe again and are ready to continue the cycle of seasons.

14 Show the rehearsed sequence to other group members.

15 Shake hands, arms, then feet to de-role.

16 Reflect on the drama.

Adaptation

1 One member from each group takes on the role of the helper who is called to help save the group.

MOVING INTO DRAMA

DRAMATIC SCENARIOS 12

Focus Co-operation, communication; making choices; whole body movement

Time 30–40 minutes

Equipment Large sticks, nytrim

Activity

1. Place sticks on the ground to form the shape of a crossroads.
2. In the large group, reflect on legends and stories about things that may happen at crossroads. Think of everyday expressions about roads and crossroads.
3. Brainstorm the kind of fictional character who might sit or stand at a crossroads to help or hinder travellers.
4. Divide into small groups of three or four people.
5. Each small group decides on the character, human or animal, who will sit or stand at the centre of their crossroads.
6. Use nytrim to reproduce the shape of their crossroads. How many roads lead into the crossroads? How large is the centre? Is there a circle of grass or other feature in the centre? Where is the crossroads?
7. The person playing the role of the character at the centre takes their place and decides on whether they will help or hinder the travellers.
8. Other members of the group are the travellers. They decide what the purpose of their journey is. Are they travelling together or separately? (If the group contains a large proportion of non-ambulant people, have wheelchairs available.)
9. Rehearse a scene which follows the following sequence:
   (a) The travellers position themselves at their starting-point.
   (b) The person at the crossroads declares who they are and why they are at the centre of the crossroads.
   (c) The travellers move slowly up the road or roads they have chosen to travel. During this time, pay attention to the way the road surface will affect movement.

MOVING INTO DRAMA

DRAMATIC SCENARIOS 12 (*Continued*)

Activity

(d) Each traveller asks the person at the centre of the crossroads for help with their journey. There are short interactions on this theme.

(e) The travellers decide whether to act on the advice given by the person at the crossroads.

(f) The travellers decide which road to take.

(g) The person at the centre makes a closing statement. The travellers make their closing statements.

10 Show the rehearsed scenes to other groups.

11 Clear away the nytrim. Member de-role by stating their own names and identifying themselves with the small group. It is important that the person who played the figure at the crossroads becomes part of the group again.

12 Return to the original crossroads of sticks and reflect on the drama. If appropriate, discuss times when group members have felt as if they were at a crossroads!

MOVING INTO DRAMA

DRAMATIC SCENARIOS 13

Focus Co-ordination, co-operation, communication and flexibility

Time 30–35 minutes

Equipment A collection of boxes of varying sizes, a large table

Activity

1. Have the boxes displayed on the table.
2. Encourage group members to examine the boxes.
3. Start to make sounds with the boxes by banging, tapping and drumming them.
4. Now imagine the boxes as wrapped presents.
5. The occasion is a visit from someone from a land far away, a place that has never been described in any book. It is a land where sound is very important. The visitor will be arriving soon and desires to know about other lands and their customs.
6. Divide into groups (which can be based on countries, counties or towns of origin or current dwelling).
7. Each group decides on the present that will be given and selects a box.
8. They decide on the characters who will be giving. Are they members of a committee, a guild or specific group? Are they a formal or informal welcome party?
9. How will the welcome party stand or sit? Groups arrange themselves around the present to form a definite shape which reflects the purpose of their group.
10. As the visitor appreciates sound, devise sounds from other boxes to welcome them.
11. Rehearse the welcoming shapes, sounds and any script that the group want to devise. (It is best to keep words to a minimum so that people do not become preoccupied with cues and remembering long speeches.)
12. Decide the order in which the groups will present and welcome.

MOVING INTO DRAMA

DRAMATIC SCENARIOS 13 (*Continued*)

Activity

13 Place a chair for the visitor in an appropriate part of the room.

14 Decide how groups will position themselves in relation to the chair. They assume these positions.

15 As the groups wait, the leader describes the entrance of the visitor. The stranger arrives. The door is opening. The visitor is standing framed by the doorway. The scent of exotic perfumes fills the room, creating a wondrous atmosphere. Slowly the visitor lifts both hands in a gesture of greeting. It is an expansive, friendly gesture which emphasizes the richness and lustre of the fabric of the visitor's clothes. Slowly, with a purposeful gait, the vistitor walks towards the chair, pleased to be here. The visitor sits and awaits the welcome.

16 In sequence, the group welcome the visitor.

17 Put the boxes back onto the table and reflect on the drama.

18 De-role with a closure exercise.

MOVING INTO DRAMA

DRAMATIC SCENARIOS 14

Focus Co-ordination, flexibility; co-operation, communication; dramatic imagination

Time 30–35 minutes

Equipment Postcards of landscapes, a large table

Conditions Physical warm-up

Activity

1 | Lay out the postcards on the table. Invite the group to look at the postcards.

2 | They choose one landscape from the selection.

3 | Using thier hands on the table surface, group members reproduce some of the shapes from the landscape.

4 | They place their elbows on the table and make shapes from the landscape using lower arms, wrists and hands.

5 | Members start to link arms, hands and wrists with others to form shapes.

6 | Move away from the table. With some people seated and some standing, group members make landscapes with their whole bodies.

7 | Add very soft sounds to the landscapes.

8 | Add movement to the sounds (trees move in the wind, mountains shake, rivers ripple). Create spaces between people.

9 | One person comes out of the shape and moves through the landscape (with or without help). Repeat, so that everyone is given a chance to move through the landscape. (Relax and rest between travellers and maybe provide more chairs so more people can sit.)

10 | Reflect on the activity.

Adaptations

1 | Landscapes in different seasons.

2 | Give the traveller an identity to form different kinds of movement.

MOVING INTO DRAMA

DRAMATIC SCENARIOS 15

Focus Communication, co-operation; imagination; hopes and wishes

Time 30 minutes

Equipment A large sheet of paper, pens

Activity

1. Brainstorm items that we make wishes with, such as blowing out candles on cakes, stars, a wishing well. Write these on the large sheet of paper.
2. Brainstorm the most common things that children wish for.
3. Divide into small groups.
4. Each small group decides on their wishing object and a child's wish.
5. In the small groups, create a drama which shows a child surrounded by a group of adults. The child mimes the actions of making a wish: for example, while stirring the Christmas pudding. The wish is made aloud. The wish is being granted. Each person is to play an active part in the drama.
6. Show these scenes to the other groups.
7. Return to the large group and reflect on the dramas and, maybe, on wishes that people have made that have been granted.

DRAMA BASED ON TEXT

POEMS

Focus Enjoyment of the rhythm of poetry; practice in reading aloud

Time 30 minutes

Equipment Copies of poems chosen for their rhythmic patterns for each group member, a table to sit around

Activity

1. Each member of the group reads as many poems as they can, silently. (If people cannot read someone else reads to them quietly.)
2. The group chooses a poem to read aloud.
3. Group members beat out the rhythm of each poem (drumming on the table) and/or use nonsense syllables to mark the rhythm (for example, la, la, la, tum-te-tum).
4. Individuals choose a poem to say aloud, enjoying the rhythm.
5. Everyone joins in to say every poem chosen (or part of it), enjoying the rhythm in unison.

Adaptations

1. The group makes up lines in the same rhythm as the verses.
2. The group concentrates on one poem, practising one kind of rhythm.

DRAMA BASED ON TEXT

POEMS ABOUT OLD AGE

Focus Reflecting upon, discussing and redefining views of old age

Time 20–30 minutes

Equipment Poems or texts about old age, such as 'Father William' from *Alice's Adventures in Wonderland; Youth and Age; King Lear*

Activity

1. Read selected extracts from a chosen text.
2. Read again.
3. Group members discuss the images that the writer is conveying.
4. What do they think of those images? Have the frustrations or joys of old age been conveyed?
5. What images do group members think that younger people have of old age?
6. Do they agree with these? How could they be changed?
7. Create a title for a play about old age. Write a speech for the play. Decide on the character who is speaking.
8. Say the speech in different ways.

Adaptations

1. Create the ideal actor to play the character making the speech.
2. Create a poster for the play saying why everyone should see it.

DRAMA BASED ON TEXT

NARRATIVE POEMS

Focus Enjoyment of poetry reading; expressing action in verse

Time 30 minutes

Equipment Copies of narrative poems, such as *The Ancient Mariner; Horatius; How they brought the Good News from Ghent to Aix; The Pied Piper of Hamelin,* for group members

Activity

1. The idea of stories in verse is introduced. The leader may read part of a poem and say how it continues and ends.
2. Members read the poem to themselves at their own speed. The leader helps those with any difficulties.
3. The group divide the poem up and read it aloud.
4. The story told by the poem is repeated, each member taking their own section and using their own words.
5. The leader reads the poem aloud and the group make actions to reflect the main events in the poem.
6. Discussion.

Adaptations

1. The whole poem is shown in mime.
2. Part of the poem may be rehearsed and spoken in unison.

DRAMA BASED ON TEXT

POETRY AND THE NATURAL WORLD

Focus How poetry increases our enjoyment of the natural world; practice in reading aloud; concentration, communication

Time 20–35 minutes

Equipment Poems about nature (Clarke, Wordsworth, Hardy, Lawrence, Blake); musical illustrations: mood music, music evoking landscapes and seascapes; music player

Activity

1. Does anyone know a poem about a winged creature? A beautiful place? Group members share memories of a poem.
2. Group leaders read aloud the prepared poems.
3. Group members are issued with copies of the prepared poems and are invited to read them.
4. Group members are encouraged to discuss the poems.
5. Group members are invited to read sections of the poems aloud.
6. The members discuss any places or events that they are reminded of by hearing the poems.
7. Group leaders play a selection of music for group members to listen to.
8. Participants match music to poems.
9. Group members are invited to read a chosen poem aloud, with music as a background to the reading.
10. The group members exchange impressions.

Adaptation

1. A poem may be chosen for speaking in unison.

DRAMA BASED ON TEXT

SHAKESPEARE 1

Focus Visualizing from a text read aloud, developing creative impulses, movement and sound; co-ordination and co-operation

Time 20–30 minutes

Activity

1. The group leader reads, slowly and clearly, the speech of Enobarbus beginning 'The barge she sat in, like a burnished throne', from Act II of *Antony and Cleopatra*.
2. The leader recaps the main images in the speech.t
3. Group members create the barge from chairs.
4. Decide who would like to play Cleopatra (this can be more than one person).
5. Position Cleopatra(s) inside the barge.
6. Members form small groups: one makes wind sounds, another makes water sounds, and the third group makes rowing movements.
7. Two groups are formed, with one or more leader per group. The first group practises Cleopatra's position, posture and bearing. How do her clothes influence her posture? What aromas will there be? The rowers practise their strokes. The second group practises wind, wave and soft crowd sounds.
8. The leader brings the two groups together. While he or she reads the speech again, the groups perform to match the reading.

DRAMA BASED ON TEXT

SHAKESPEARE 2

Focus Views of old age, conflicts between youth and age; movement, working with creative impulses, co-operation

Time 30–40 minutes

Equipment None

Conditions Physical warm-up

Activity

1. The leaders set the scene for Polonius's speech to his son in Act I, Scene III of *Hamlet*.
2. Two leaders read the scene with some prepared movement (amend as necessary to fit in with the group's concentration span). The movement should serve to highlight the father/son relationship.
3. Group members are encouraged to discuss their perceptions of the way Polonius's age and Laertes's youth influence their relationship.
4. The leaders invite suggestions for bringing the scene into the twentieth century.
5. In pairs, group members devise short improvisations on the theme of the old giving sound advice to the young.
6. They share the improvisations.
7. All reflect on the presented dramas.

DRAMA BASED ON TEXT

SHAKESPEARE 3

Focus Youth and age, changing stereotypes; creative impulses; movement, co-ordination and co-operation

Time 30–40 minutes

Equipment None

Conditions Physical warm-up

Activity

1. Set the scene for *Romeo and Juliet*, Act II, Scene 5. The leader tells the story of Romeo and Juliet.
2. Leaders perform a rehearsed reading of the scene.
3. What issues about the relationship between Juliet and the nurse do group members feel are raised by the scene?
4. How would the scene be if the nurse was in love and waiting for Juliet to bring her news?
5. In pairs, members prepare short improvisations, set in the present, that portray an elderly person in love and waiting for news to be brought to them by a young person.
6. Pairs share their improvisations in turn, after which the whole group comments upon them.

DRAMA BASED ON TEXT

SHAKESPEARE 4

Focus Redefining negative views of old age

Time 20–30 minutes

Equipment Copies of Jaques's speech beginning 'All the world's a stage' from Act II of *As You Like It*, pens and paper

Activity

1. The group leader reads the whole speech in a clear voice.
2. Repeat from 'Last scene of all...'
3. Ask for the group's views on this. Point out that Jaques is represented as a homespun philosopher with a slightly embittered and ironical view of life.
4. If Jaques were taking a different view of life, how might the final line 'Sans teeth, sans eyes, sans taste, sans everything' be changed? Ask group members to reword the line, replacing the 'sans' (without) with the word 'with' and saying what is still present in old age.
5. Members share their reworked lines.

DRAMA BASED ON TEXT

FAIRY TALES 1

Focus Revising known stories; using the imagination; group co-operation

Time 20–30 minutes

Equipment None

Conditions Physical warm-up

Activity

1. Group leaders have devised a short (three-minute) scene from a fairy story: for example, Cinderella trying on the slipper. One player should be seated, while the other moves about. They show their scene in such a position that they can be seen and heard by all the group members.
2. They repeat the scene with roles reversed.
3. The group recalls the whole story.
4. In pairs, group members create their own version of the scene.
5. The group members show the scene they have devised.

DRAMA BASED ON TEXT

FAIRY TALES 2

Focus Images of old age; creativity; reworking of experience

Time 25–35 minutes

Equipment Pens and paper

Activity

1. The group leader recounts the story of Red Riding Hood.
2. Focus on grandmother's cottage (male group members may want to change the character to a grandfather).
3. What characteristics does grandmother have?
4. Draw a picture of grandmother's cottage in the forest.
5. What is this person's relationship with Red Riding Hood's parents?
6. How does grandmother live each day? How is she self-sufficient?
7. Focus on the visit from the wolf.
8. How could the character defeat the wolf?
9. In pairs, group members create a strategy to defeat the wolf.
10. They share their strategies.
11. Discuss the strategies and how effective they could be.

DRAMA BASED ON TEXT

FAIRY TALES 3

Focus Stereotypes and childhood views of old age; creative impulses

Time 20–30 minutes

Equipment Large sheets of paper and felt-tip pens

Conditions Physical warm-up

Activity

1. Brainstorm onto a large sheet of paper titles of fairy or folk tales.
2. On another sheet of paper, write the names of all the old people in the stories.
3. Divide these into wise old people and wicked old people and write them on separate sheets.
4. Create two groups: one leader per group, one group for each sheet of paper.
5. Group members focus on the body and create shapes to represent the two views of old people: one group as the wise old people and one group as the wicked old people!
6. Each group prepares a very short statement about themselves: one group about their wisdom, the other about how they enjoy creating havoc.
7. The groups share the shapes and statements with each other.
8. Group discussion on the drama.

DRAMA BASED ON TEXT

NEWSPAPERS 1

Focus Social awareness, movement, creativity

Time 30–35 minutes

Equipment Newspaper articles reporting two contrasting events: for example, news about homeless people and about the lavish lifestyle of other people

Conditions Physical warm-up

Activity

1 Leaders read newspaper articles aloud.

2 The group discuss the differences and give their opinions.

3 Divide members into two groups, with one leader per group. Devise a short drama or improvisation that shows the differences between the two situations described in the article.

4 Discuss the dramas and the social issues raised in them.

DRAMA BASED ON TEXT

NEWSPAPERS 2

Focus To engage in discussion; movement and creative impulses; co-operation

Time 30–35 minutes

Equipment Flip chart, newspaper articles describing a particular event of national interest (serious or fun)

Conditions Physical warm-up

Activity

1. Leaders read the articles aloud.
2. The main facts are written on the flip chart.
3. Identify the main people involved.
4. What do group members think of them?
5. Define the main physical and psychological characteristics of these people.
6. Group leaders call out the names of the people involved in the news items. Group members reproduce the stance and characteristics of the person whose name has been called.
7. People choose a person from the news items to play (try to negotiate the same number of people to play each person). Depending on the news item, some people may be part of a crowd.
8. In small groups, members prepare short scenarios that portray the news event.
9. Discuss.

DRAMA BASED ON TEXT

NEWSPAPERS 3

Focus Debate; political issues; formulating and voicing opinions

Time 30–35 minutes

Equipment Articles from different newspapers about issues that affect the elderly, main points from these on a flip chart

Conditions Physical warm-up

Activity

1. Introduce the topic.
2. Leaders read the articles aloud.
3. Leaders and group members together outline the main points and highlight the different perspectives given by the newspapers.
4. Debate the main issues.
5. In pairs or threes, members devise short scenes to illustrate the possible consequences of legislation: for example, the consequences of VAT on fuel or the issues of free bus travel.
6. Discuss the improvisations.

PUPPETS, MASKS AND CELEBRATION

A WORD OF CAUTION

Focus It should always be remembered that masks and puppets are a very powerful means of making things dramatic — so powerful, indeed, that they seem to have a life of their own. If you are an imaginative sort of person, you can actually feel the masks at work trying to take over and make you behave like them. It is a good idea to be aware of this, as it often makes the unwary feel very uncomfortable.

This experience of being taken out of yourself by the role you are playing belongs to another kind of dramatherapy, however. Here we are focusing on masks as a story-telling aid. The idea is to celebrate what we know and enjoy rather than to reveal things that were hidden from us.

Items needed Thick card of various colours and thicknesses. Bamboo canes of various shapes and sizes. Nets of different colours and textures. Hollow balls (polystyrene, plastic footballs and so on). Clothing, fabric pieces and scraps. Glue, scissors, rulers, staples and brushes.

Paints, felt-tip pens, glitter, spray silver and gold paints, beads and lace.

Items such as old table tennis bats, soft cane wicker backings for wall flower arrangements; cardboard circles from frozen food containers and circular foil containers can make useful mask bases.

PUPPETS, MASKS AND CELEBRATION

GROUPMASK 1

Focus Creativity; movement; self-affirmation, expression of feeling

Time 30–35 minutes

Equipment A 'lost' mask: upset and needing help (this may be influenced by a feeling of being unhappy expressed, during other groups, by group members), mask-making equipment, a large table

Conditions Physical warm-up

Activity

1. Show group members the ready-made 'lost' mask.
2. The group decide how and why this mask is 'lost'.
3. What help does the mask need?
4. The group make the 'helper' mask.
5. Put this mask where everyone can see it.
6. What kind of help can each group member contribute to the 'lost' mask?
7. Group members mime the helping movement.
8. Create the story of the 'lost' mask being helped by the 'helper' mask.
9. How does the 'lost' mask look when it has been helped?
10. Create this other mask celebrating the change in the 'lost' mask.
11. Reflect on the story.
12. What will group members do with the masks?

PUPPETS, MASKS AND CELEBRATION

GROUPMASK 2

Focus Creativity, self-affirmation (group and individual)

Time 30–35 minutes

Equipment Mask-making equipment, pens and paper, a large table and flip chart

Activity

1. Each person has a pen and paper.
2. They write down three aspects of themselves that they are proud of, such as strength, persistence, kindness, generosity and compassion.
3. If anyone is unable to think of three qualities, allow suggestions from other group members.
4. Write all the qualities on the flip chart.
5. What kind of mask would have these qualities?
6. Draw an outline of the mask and cut out.
7. The group make the mask.
8. Place the completed mask where everyone can see it.
9. Looking at the mask, group members decide what is the collective strength of this group.
10. Discuss what each individual can give to and take from this collective strength.

PUPPETS, MASKS AND CELEBRATION

GROUPMASK 3

Focus Creativity; co-operation; movement; self-affirmation

Time 30–40 minutes

Equipment Mask-making equipment, pens and paper, a large table.

Conditions Physical warm-up

Activity

1 On a large sheet of paper the group brainstorm fictional heroes and heroines.

2 Favourites are identified.

3 On a round sheet of paper, the group brainstorm their favourites' good qualities.

4 How are these qualities shown, physically, in their face (big, wide eyes, straight nose)? Which physical attributes do we connect with honesty (or dishonesty)?

5 Negotiate with the group about the colour and shape of the mask.

6 Draw an outline on card and cut it out.

7 Decorate the mask, to make it a hero's mask.

8 Put the completed mask where everyone can see it.

9 Ask what kind of posture this person would have.

10 The group assume postures, making them large and expansive.

11 Create movement from these postures.

12 Holding the mask in front of their body, individuals can relate to times when they were a hero or heroine. As they recount their story, they take up a hero/heroine posture. (If people are unable to hold the mask, the group leader holds it in front of their body.)

NB The mask should not be in front of the face, as this will muffle the voice and create a different dimension to the activity which has not been prepared for.

13 Discuss and decide what group members want to do with the mask.

PUPPETS, MASKS AND CELEBRATION

GROUPMASK 4

Focus Awareness of the season; creativity; celebrating self and culture

Time 30–40 minutes

Equipment A large table, thick card, paints, glitter, fabric, lace, pens, paper, scissors, glue, stapler and staples

Activity

1. Talk about the special day that you are approaching. (This could be Christmas, Easter, Halloween and so on, or a special day from other cultures that group members may come from.)
2. Brainstorm and write down items and people connected with this day. (For example, 5 November: bonfire, fireworks, toffee apples, baked potatoes, guys.)
3. On another sheet of paper, group members write the colours that are connected with the above (they write, for example, the word 'brown' in brown felt-tip).
4. Tell the group that you are going to make a mask for the day.
5. Ask for suggestions about the shape of the mask.
6. Draw an outline for a large mask on card and cut it out.
7. What do the group want on the mask (colours, design and so on)?
8. Lay chosen items onto the mask to see how they look before securing them.
9. When the mask is completed, allow and encourage members to hold it.
10. Put the mask in a place where everyone can see it.
11. Allowing the mask to influence colours and shapes, each person makes a card for the group, with a celebratory message relating to the day.
12. Group members share their cards and then place them around the mask to create a group celebration.
13. What do the group want to do with the mask and cards?

Adaptation

1. If group members are from different cultures, dedicate different group sessions to different cultures.

GROUPMASK 5

Focus Overview of a situation; movement; creative impulses

Time 30–35 minutes

Equipment Mask-making equipment, feathers, postcards of birds, a table

Conditions Physical warm-up

Activity

1 Display postcards for group members to look at.

2 Discuss the birds shown and their characteristics.

3 Make a bird mask.

4 Put the mask where everyone can see it.

5 Group members decide how this bird would perch. How would the body and head be? They make these movements. How would this bird preen itself? They make the movement. How would it splash in water? They make the movement. What movements would it make when eating? They make these movements.

6 Decide on a short journey this bird might make.

7 During the bird's journey it will see a difficult situation involving humans: what is this situation?

8 Group members make the movements of the bird preparing for the journey and setting out. They make the movements of gliding and flying in the wind. Suddenly the bird has an overview of the situation involving the humans.

9 Group members make the movement of the bird, alighting to rest and watching.

10 The bird decides to take the situation to a counsel of birds.

11 Group members become the council of birds and give advice.

12 The bird flies away to tell the humans. Members make the movement of flying.

PUPPETS, MASKS AND CELEBRATION

GROUPMASK 5 (*Continued*)

Activity

13 The group, as themselves, decide how the bird will tell the humans the counsel's advice.

14 The group reflect on what has happened in the session.

15 Decide what to do with the mask.

PUPPETS, MASKS AND CELEBRATION

GROUPMASK 6

Focus Sensory perceptions; movement; creativity

Time 30–35 minutes

Equipment Mask-making equipment, perfume sprays that can be squirted into the air

Conditions Physical warm-up

Activity

1. Discuss scents and how some celebrations are connected with them.
2. Spray some of the scents into the air near people and let them smell. Perhaps have some large, easily handled objects, such as an orange with a clove stuck into it, for people to smell.
3. Ask about images that are connected with these perfumes. Discuss.
4. What are the most popular scents? Reduce these to one group favourite.
5. Smell this scent again and think of the kind of atmosphere of celebration it evokes.
6. Describe the atmosphere in detail.
7. What kind of person may exist in this atmosphere? What are they celebrating?
8. Make the mask of the person.
9. Decide how this person will move. Group members make these movements.
10. What is the ritual of the celebration? The group create the ritual.
11. The group reflect upon the activity.
12. They decide what to do with the mask.

PUPPETS, MASKS AND CELEBRATION

GROUPMASK 7

Focus Self-affirmation; creativity, movements

Time 30–35 minutes

Equipment Mask-making equipment, a large table, pens and paper

Conditions Physical warm-up

Activity

1. Ask group members to think about important people in public life.
2. What makes them important?
3. How do they make themselves look important?
4. Group members take on the postures and facial expressions of very important people.
5. They create the mask of a very important person (not an actual person, but a representative mask).
6. How would the body of this mask move? Group members reproduce these movements.
7. How do important people greet others? Does feeling important change their reactions to others? Group members move as if they think other people are unimportant. They greet others as if they think they are important.
8. Think about ways in which other people in the group are important.
9. Each group member writes a short note to others to tell them why they are important.
10. They deliver the notes.
11. They read them out.
12. Group members write a note to themselves to say why they are important and how they can celebrate being important (the leader may need to prompt).
13. Group members share thoughts and feelings.
14. Decide what to do with the mask.

PUPPETS, MASKS AND CELEBRATION

GROUPMASK 8

Focus Self-expression; movement; creative impulses

Time 30–35 minutes

Equipment Postcards of land and sea, mask-making equipment, a large table

Conditions Physical warm-up

Activity

1. The group look at the postcards of land and sea; discuss them.
2. They discuss movements and then make them: trees and plants (stretching upwards); rain and water (stretching and reaching down); wind (shifting sideways, stretching) and so on. Flowing tide (gentle swaying); stormy sea (faster upwards movement); ebbing tide (flowing inward movement) and so on.
3. Divide the group into two.
4. Make land and sea masks: one for each group.
5. In the two groups, members devise movements and add soft sounds (they should not make loud sounds, which could strain the voice).
6. They add the sets of movement together and devise a land and sea movement sequence.
7. The two masks are put together and the group discuss how they complement each other.
8. Members reflect on groupwork and masks.
9. They decide what to do with the masks.

PUPPETS, MASKS AND CELEBRATION

PUPPETS 1

Focus Expressing desires; co-ordination, group cohesion, co-operation

Time 30–40 minutes

Equipment A large stick in a secure base, green fabric (quilts, for example), tinsel or similar, shiny paper, Christmas tree decorations (if available), fairy doll (or puppet) or large star, large safety pins

Activity

1. Think about Christmas and when and where you can make wishes.
2. Suggest that one place for making wishes is by the star or fairy at the top of a Christmas tree.
3. Make a Christmas tree by draping the green fabric across the top of the pole and creating shapes.
4. Decorate the tree by pinning decorations to it.
5. Group members make a star, or a doll into a moving puppet, which can grant children's wishes.
6. Group members take it in turns to be the puppet manipulator.
7. The puppet hears wishes and moves in response to each one. (Group members make wishes as children at Christmas: the leader should encourage child-like (not childish) movements.)
8. When everyone has taken part who wishes to, dismantle the tree.
9. Members reflect on how it felt to ask and how it was to be the puppeteer. The leader may want to address whether asking for what you want is the privilege of children.
10. Close with a thank you to the granters of wishes.

PUPPETS, MASKS AND CELEBRATION

PUPPETS 2

Focus Hand movement; co-operation, communication, co-ordination; creativity

Time 30–40 minutes

Equipment Celebration music, paper cups (a few already made into faces), staples, coloured paper or coloured tissue paper, a table

Conditions Warmed-up hands

Activity

1. Have paper cups upside-down on the table, arranged in a circle.
2. Ask people to move the cups, making sounds with them.
3. Group members hold one cup and imagine what is in it. They make drinking movements.
4. What would be in the cups for a celebration?
5. Group members empty the cup and turn it upside-down.
6. They imagine characters who might celebrate by having a drink, and describe them.
7. The leader shows the cups already made into faces and asks group members to make their own, by stapling paper to their cups.
8. When everyone has finished, they put their paper cups on their hands.
9. The leader plays the music and group members respond with their paper cup puppet. Relax.
10. The leader changes the music to something with a faster beat. The puppets move again.
11. Some puppets are getting a bit drunk. Members show this in movement. (People who decline to have their puppet drunk can show how the puppet responds to those who are.)
12. Slower music is played: the puppets are becoming tired, their movements become slower.

PUPPETS, MASKS AND CELEBRATION

PUPPETS 2 (*Continued*)

Activity

13 The puppets go to sleep.

14 Group members slip their hands out of their cups.

15 They shake their hands.

16 They put their puppets onto the table and say goodbye.

17 The group reflect on the celebration.

18 They decide what to do with the puppets.

PUPPETS, MASKS AND CELEBRATION

PUPPETS 3

Focus Dramatic creativity; hand movement; co-operation, co-ordination

Time 30–40 minutes

Equipment A sheet suspended between two bases (high enough for two people to go behind without being seen), a selection of toys (preferably the kind of cuddly toys that some adults like — other staff may be willing to lend these)

Conditions Warmed-up arms, shoulders and hands

Activity

1. Have the toys on the table for people to pick up as they choose. Do not impose touching: encourage rather than tell. Talk about the toys.
2. Ask about the textures and colours.
3. Ask people to choose one toy (people who do not wish to do so should be allowed to decline).
4. Group members make movements with the toys. Those without toys are to watch, to be the audience.
5. Group members decide on a character for each toy.
6. Members are divided into small groups. Include people without toys in groups with toys.
7. Group members create a short scenario in which the toys are characters. Those without toys should be encouraged to join in with ideas.
8. Holding the toys in the air, members enact the scene. (If anyone cannot lift their arms, the group leader can hold the toy and the group member provide the voice.)
9. Short performances of these scenes are given, with puppeteers going behind the sheet to move the toys.
10. Show all the performances. (Make these very visual, as some people may not be able to hear. Arrange seating so that those without sight or with impaired sight are very close. The group leader may sit near them and repeat any dialogue.)
11. The group discuss the performances and celebrate the group as performers and script creators.

PUPPETS, MASKS AND CELEBRATION

PUPPETS 4

Focus Co-operation; dramatic imagination; self-affirmation

Time 30–40 minutes

Equipment A bamboo stick set firmly on a base, with another stick secured in a horizontal position for arms and a ball securely fixed to the top of the stick as a head, assorted scissors and fabrics

Conditions Warmed-up arms, shoulders and hands

Activity

1. Put the puppet base in the centre of the group so the group members can all see.
2. Group members feel the fabrics, stroking, touching and pulling.
3. The plan is to make a celebration puppet: to turn this base into a celebration.
4. Ask what the group want to celebrate. Reach an agreement about the celebration.
5. Start to put a face on the ball (group members may do this or instruct the leader).
6. Add hair and hat.
7. Drape fabric to make clothing.
8. Look at the puppet from different places in the room.
9. The group pose for a photograph by the puppet, creating an image of group celebration. (Group leaders may actually take a photograph or mime.)
10. Where will people put the photograph (real or imagined)?
11. Dismantle the puppet or decide where to keep it.
12. Reflect on the session.

PUPPETS, MASKS AND CELEBRATION

PUPPETS 5

Focus Hand movement, flexibility; creativity, communication

Time 30–35 minutes

Equipment One brightly coloured sock per person

Conditions Hands warmed up

Activity

1. Group members move their hands into different shapes.
2. They shake their hands to release any tension.
3. Make animal shapes with hands: birds pecking, fish swimming, birds flying, and so on.
4. In small groups, members interact with each other using hands only.
5. Group leader displays the socks and asks people to try some on their hands and move their hands about. Does the colour of the sock suggest different movements?
6. Decide on one sock per person.
7. Participants make hand movements.
8. Decide on the kind of character the movement and colour suggest: for example, Jack-in-the-box, other toys, animals and birds.
9. Group members develop movement in relation to their puppet's character.
10. The puppet characters interact with one another. Relax.
11. Add words to the interaction. Relax.
12. Think about a celebration the puppets might share.
13. Show the puppets celebrating. Relax (maybe with some music).
14. Members resume celebrating and let their free hands mirror the movements of the hands with the puppets, or come close to them.

PUPPETS, MASKS AND CELEBRATION

PUPPETS 5 (*Continued*)

Activity

15 Puppets say good-bye to each other.

16 Members take off the socks and say good-bye to the character.

PUPPETS 6

Focus Celebration of self; imagination, creativity

Time 30–35 minutes

Equipment Fabrics suitable for making a wizard, hats, gloves, wool for hair, an assortment of material

Conditions Physical warm-up

Activity

1. Put a large bamboo cane, mop handle or stick on the floor in the middle of the group. Place a large ball at one end for the head.
2. Tell the story of *The Wizard of Oz* (3 minutes maximum).
3. The group recap the main points.
4. Make the objects on the floor into the Wizard of Oz. (The puppet will not be moved, so items do not need to be secured.)
5. Try several ways of creating the wizard. (Group leaders may need to actually place items following instructions of group members.)
6. Divide members into a scarecrow group, a lion group and a tin man/woman group.
7. Recap on what each group wants from the wizard.
8. Groups experiment with movement of their chosen character.
9. Each group, making appropriate movements, asks the wizard for what they want (no answer from the wizard).
10. On receiving no answer, each group discovers that they have what they want anyway (a heart, a brain and courage). How have they discovered this? People can stick to the story or make up their own reasons.
11. How did it feel for group members to discover that they have these qualities anyway?
12. Reflect on the drama.
13. Dismantle the wizard, then comment on him.

CLOSURES

MOVEMENT 1

Focus Preparing for leaving, good-byes

Time 10 minutes

Equipment None

Activity

1. Group members imagine a very large cake on a table where everyone can see it.
2. The cake has many candles.
3. Group members blow out the candles.
4. It is too late to eat the cake. Each person takes a piece and wraps it up to take away.
5. People thank each other for the cake and say good-bye. Maybe they would enjoy some cake this evening. (The cake has, of course, been baked to cater for every diet.)

CLOSURES

MOVEMENT 2

Focus Preparing for leaving, good-byes

Time 10 minutes

Equipment None

Activity

1. Group members sit well back in their chairs, with hands on thighs.
2. They stretch and relax their hands. Repeat three times.
3. Divide the group into messengers and senders.
4. Messengers go to senders and receive a handshake and a good-bye.
5. Senders give messengers a handshake for other senders. Messengers deliver. Messengers also give each other handshakes.

CLOSURES

MOVEMENT 3

Focus Preparing for leaving, good-byes

Time 10 minutes

Equipment A ball of nytrim or string

Activity

1. Use nytrim or string to pass round the group, each person holding it. The group leader may need to help. The group does not need to be in a circle. The nytrim or string should be quite slack.
2. The group leader holds the ball of nytrim or string.
3. Members move the nytrim or string different distances away, up and down.
4. All together, they make good-bye statements and drop the nytrium or string.
5. When no-one is holding the nytrim or string and it is all on the floor, the group leader rewinds the ball.

CLOSURES

MOVEMENT 4

Focus Relaxing and unwinding before leaving the group

Time 10 minutes

Equipment None

Activity

1. The group members sit well back into their chairs, have hands on thighs, hands and legs uncrossed.
2. They breathe slowly and deeply, not holding their breath or slowing down their breathing.
3. They let their bodies relax.
4. Slowly they bring their hands into a soft movement, a flowing wave.
5. They wave good-bye to other members of the group.
6. They breathe deeply as they prepare to move from the room.
7. Any last waves?
8. They say good-bye to the people nearest to them.

CLOSURES

MOVEMENT 5

Focus Preparing for leaving

Time 10 minutes

Equipment None

Activity

1. Sit well back in your chair.
2. Move your feet and legs or move your body slightly forward.
3. On the spot move your feet in walking movements or move your body backwards and forwards (maybe only a fraction.)
4. Imagine yourself leaving the room.
5. What thoughts or feelings will you be taking with you?
6. Share some of these with others.
7. Say good-bye to others in the group.

CLOSURES

MOVEMENT 6

Focus Closing a session, deroling from a character

Time 10–15 minutes

Equipment None

Activity

1. Think of a character.
2. Imagine you have a large crystal ball in your hands or on your lap.
3. Look into the ball and see the character waving good-bye, going on a long journey. The character becomes smaller and smaller as they retreat into the distance. Mentally wave good-bye.
4. Put down the crystal ball.
5. Tell the other group members that the character has gone; say why you enjoyed meeting them.
6. When everyone has spoken, make waving gestures of good-bye to the character.
7. Focus on other people in the group. Wave good-bye to them. Initiate and return waves.

CLOSURES

MOVEMENT 7

Focus Closing a session, deroling from a character

Time 10–15 minutes

Equipment None

Activity

1. Think of a character.
2. What did you like about the character?
3. What did you dislike?
4. Imagine you can pick up the bits you did not like. Put them in the centre of the room or away from you and ask someone to put them in the centre.
5. When all these bits have been collected, imagine them as a bonfire and light it. Warm your hands at the flames.
6. Imagine throwing buckets of water on the fire until it is out.
7. Say why you are glad those bits have gone.
8. Say good-bye to the others in the group.

CLOSURES

MOVEMENT 8

Focus Closing a session, deroling from a character

Time 10–15 minutes

Equipment None

Activity

1. Imagine you have a large jar in front of you.
2. Think about the character you have been playing.
3. Decide on things about the character you do not want.
4. Mime putting these in the jar.
5. Mime sealing the jar.
6. Mime putting it on a shelf.
7. Tell others about your jar. Say your name.
8. Say good-bye to others in the group.

CLOSURES

MOVEMENT 9

Focus Closing a session, deroling from a character

Time 10–15 minutes

Equipment None

Activity

1. Take up the posture of your character.
2. Imagine you are holding a feather duster.
3. Brush your body with the duster. As you do this you imagine you are brushing off bits of the character you do not want.
4. Brush these bits onto the floor.
5. Imagine you have a large brush; sweep these bits away.
6. Notice other people in the group.
7. Say good-bye and give them a kind thought for the rest of the day.

CLOSURES

MOVEMENT 10

Focus Ending a group, deroling from a character

Time 10–15 minutes

Equipment Pens and paper

Activity

1. Make a movement you have enjoyed making as the character.
2. Enlarge this movement.
3. Change the movement.
4. Make a movement that the character enabled you to do today.
5. Repeat the movement.
6. Write a note, such as 'I, Jane Smythe, thank the lion for the movement of beating my chest — this is my movement now.' (Some people may need help.)
7. Show others the movement, saying your own name.
8. Make a good-bye movement as yourself.

CLOSURES

MOVEMENT 11

Focus Saying good-bye, relaxing, leaving the group

Time 10 minutes

Equipment Soft, relaxing music and music player

Activity

1. Group members sit well back in their chairs.
2. Play the music and suggest that members listen and relax.
3. As they relax, ask them to look around the group at other people relaxing.
4. They make small head movements to the music.
5. With these head movements only, they nod good-bye to others in the group.
6. They smile at people and return their good-byes with small, relaxed waves.
7. Turn off the music and ask group members to slowly make their bodies alert for leaving.
8. They make any further good-byes.

CLOSURES

MOVEMENT 12

Focus Leaving the group, saying good-bye, relaxing

Time 10 minutes

Equipment None

Activity

1. Sit well back in your chairs.
2. Imagine the chair is huge and soft. You are very, very comfortable. You do not want to move.
3. Now imagine the chair is even more comfortable. Relax into it.
4. As you relax, recall all the things you have done in the group today.
5. Remember other people and the things you have enjoyed seeing them doing.
6. Turn your attention to them.
7. Your hands want to move. Let your hands and arms make small mimes of some of the things you have enjoyed seeing others doing.
8. The rest of you wants to move. Show some others the mimes you have just done.
9. Thank others for letting you share these things.
10. Say good-byes.

CLOSURES

MOVEMENT 13

Focus Saying good-bye, deroling from character

Time 10 minutes

Equipment None

Activity

1. Focus on the character you have played today.
2. Make a movement that the character made.
3. Make the movement bigger.
4. Stretch and let the character leave your body. Stretch again and relax.
5. Breathe deeply and really become aware of your own body.
6. Stretch and relax.
7. Look at other group members.
8. Stretch again and turn the stretch into a wave to others.
9. Say good-byes.

CLOSURES

MOVEMENT 14

Focus Saying good-bye, deroling

Time 10 minutes

Equipment None

Activity

1. Think about the character you have played.
2. Imagine that running at your feet is a clear, beautiful stream.
3. Become clear about the aspects of the character that you do not want to keep.
4. Imagine that you can roll these aspects up in your hand. Make the hand movements.
5. Drop the rolled items into the stream and watch them float away.
6. The stream dries up.
7. Notice other people in the room.
8. Say good-bye to each person.

CLOSURES

MOVEMENT 15

Focus Saying good-bye

Time 15 minutes

Equipment A collection of hats, a large table

Activity

1. Have the hats on the table.
2. Group members sit around the table.
3. They look at the hats.
4. They try some on, keeping one.
5. How might a person wearing this hat say good-bye?
6. Group members say good-bye in the manner of this person.
7. They change hats and repeat.
8. They change hats and repeat.
9. They return the hats to the table.
10. They say good-bye as themselves, repeating several times.
11. They say good-bye as themselves, with a statement about themselves in today's group.

CLOSURES

MOVEMENT 16

Focus Saying good-bye

Time 10 minutes

Equipment None

Activity

1. Each group member thinks of themselves as a famous actor.
2. They imagine that they have all just given the most wonderful performances.
3. They get into postures.
4. They start by blowing kisses of congratulation to each other.
5. They introduce superlatives, such as 'super', 'wonderful', 'fabulous'.
6. They start with and add endearments, such as 'darling', 'lovey', 'sweetie'.
7. They make huge gestures, exaggerated congratulations.
8. Group members revert to themselves.
9. They offer sincere congratulations to other group members for their creativity in the group.
10. They say good-byes.

CLOSURES

MOVEMENT 17

Focus Saying good-bye

Time 10 minutes

Equipment Music with a marked beat, music player

Activity

1. The leader starts a clapping rhythm.
2. Group members join in the rhythm.
3. Music is played; they clap to the beat of the rhythm.
4. They continue clapping to the rhythm, with the hand against any surface other than the other hand.
5. The music is turned off.
6. Group members find a clapping rhythm to 'good-bye'.
7. They clap 'good-bye'.
8. They clap to 'farewell'.
9. They say good-bye.

CLOSURES

MOVEMENT 18

Focus Saying good-bye

Time 10 minutes

Equipment None

Activity

1. Brainstorm ways of saying 'hello' in different cultures.
2. Perform some of these, with some people still and some moving.
3. Brainstorm ways of saying 'good-bye' in different cultures.
4. Perform these as good-byes for today.

CLOSURES

MOVEMENT 19

Focus Saying good-bye to other group members

Time 10 minutes

Equipment A large table

Activity

1. The group sits around a large table.
2. They imagine that there is a large tea pot on the table, with milk, sugar and cakes.
3. They imagine that everyone has a special cup in front of them.
4. They mime pouring tea and milk, adding sugar, passing cakes.
5. They mime eating and drinking.
6. The group leader announces that it is nearly time to go.
7. Everyone mimes pushing cups into the centre of the table.
8. They reflect on the fact that cups of tea are a good end to things in general.
9. They say good-byes.

CLOSURES

MOVEMENT 20

Focus Good-byes and wishes for other group members

Time 10 minutes

Equipment None

Activity

1. Everyone sits comfortably.
2. They imagine that in the centre of the room is a large wishing well.
3. Some group members move to turn the handle and bring up a bucket. Those seated clap a rhythm for them to move to. (The group leader may need to suggest a rhythm.)
4. When the group decides that the bucket is up and secure, everyone sits.
5. Each person prepares a wish for the group or for specific group members.
6. Wishes are placed carefully in the bucket and the bucket is lowered, to a different rhythm.
7. Group members reflect on the wishes.
8. They say their thanks and good-byes.

CLOSURES

MOVEMENT 21

Focus Deroling, saying good-bye

Time 10 minutes

Equipment None

Activity

1. Sit well back in your chair.
2. Close your eyes and imagine that it is a hot, sunny day. Breathe deeply and imagine that you are in a beautiful garden. Imagine the character you have just played walking in the garden. See the character smelling the flowers. They eventually stop at one flowerbed and pick a flower. You see the character smiling at you. They offer a flower to you and you take it. It is given as a good-bye. Hold the flower in your hands. The character waves good-bye and you watch them go.
3. Open your eyes. Move your hands as if holding the flower.
4. Show the flower to others in the group. Describe it.
5. Say good-bye to others in the group.

CLOSURES

MOVEMENT 22

Focus Saying good-bye, leaving the group, taking something away from the group

Time 10 minutes

Equipment None

Activity

1. Sit well back in your chair.
2. Relax—have your feet firmly on the ground.
3. Breathe deeply and reflect on the group.
4. Imagine that in front of you are three caskets: one gold, one silver and one glass.
5. Imagine that there is something from today's group in each one.
6. Take something from each casket — reach out your hand and take it. You may not know what it will be before you reach out.
7. Place these things on your lap, very carefully.
8. Share with others the things you have found.
9. Thank others for enabling you to collect these items.
10. Say good-byes.

CLOSURES

GOOD-BYES AND GIFTS 1

Focus Leaving the group; positive thoughts for others and self

Time 10 minutes

Equipment A large sheet of paper, pens

Activity

1. The group leader asks participants to reflect on the smiles they have seen in the group today. They may have only been there for a short while but should be remembered.
2. Each person draws a smile on the paper in front of them, making these quite large.
3. Members present their drawn smiles to others in the group. They say why they would like to give them to other people in the group.
4. Each person smiles as they finish speaking.
5. They say good-byes.

CLOSURES

GOOD-BYES AND GIFTS 2

Focus Leaving the group, good-byes; what happens next

Time 10 minutes

Equipment A large table, pens and paper

Activity

1. Think about the time.
2. What will you be doing next?
3. How will the activity you do next be influenced by what you have been doing now?
4. Draw your journey to the next place you will be in.
5. Share these journeys.
6. Share any positive thoughts about people in the group that you will be taking with you.
7. Say good-bye to others in the group.

CLOSURES

GOOD-BYES AND GIFTS 3

Focus Leaving with a positive statement about self and group; sharing thoughts about others

Time 10 minutes

Equipment A large sheet of paper, pens, a large table

Activity

1. Group members sit around the table.
2. On the large sheet of paper, each person writes their name.
3. Around their name they write the names of the other people in the group.
4. Around these, to enclose all the names, each person draws a circle. They turn this circle into a symbol of a good feeling about themselves and the group (for example, a sun, a star, a bracelet).
5. People share their symbols.
6. They say good-byes.

CLOSURES

GOOD-BYES AND GIFTS 4

Focus Leaving with a gift from others

Time 10 minutes

Equipment Postcards, a large table

Activity

1. Postcards are spread out on the table that the group are sitting around.
2. People look at the postcards.
3. The group leader tells them to choose a postcard for themselves and one for each of the other group members.
4. They decide why they want to send postcards to others.
5. Group leaders act as deliverers.
6. Postcards are sent with verbal messages between group members.
7. When deliveries are completed, people look at their collection and say why they are pleased to receive them.
8. They focus on why they have given themselves the card they chose and say why they are pleased to have it.
9. What will people do with the cards?
10. They say their good-byes and thank-yous.

CLOSURES

GOOD-BYES AND GIFTS 5

Focus Leaving the group, good-byes, deroling

Time 10 minutes

Equipment Pens and paper

Activity

1. Group members think about the character they have been playing.
2. They fold an A4 sheet of paper in half. On one side, they write a short good-bye to the character. On the other, they state what they have learned from the character. They create a gift for the character, which they draw.
3. Group members show the gift picture and state why they want to give this character a good-bye gift.
4. They create, on paper, a gift for themselves.
5. They tell other group members what the gift is.
6. Group members tell others that they deserve the gift.
7. They say their good-byes and thanks.

CLOSURES

GOOD-BYES AND GIFTS 6

Focus Saying good-bye

Time 10 minutes

Equipment Song sheets

Activity

1. Think about songs that have 'good-bye' as the main theme.
2. Brainstorm these.
3. Sing a few bars of some of them.
4. Hand out song sheets you have prepared.
5. Led by the group leaders, group members clap the rhythm.
6. Everyone sings and claps to the songs.
7. They say good-bye.

CLOSURES

GOOD-BYES AND GIFTS 7

Focus Saying good-bye and accepting gifts

Time 10 minutes

Equipment A large table

Activity

1. Group members sit around the table.
2. They imagine that in the centre of the table is a large candle.
3. They decide on the colour of the candle. What symbolism does this colour have for the group?
4. Each person imagines that they have a smaller candle of the same colour in front of them.
5. Someone mimes lighting the large candle.
6. Each person mimes lighting a taper from the large candle and lighting their own, stating what they are taking from the large candle for themselves.
7. They all sit and reflect for a while.
8. They mime blowing out the small candles and then the large one.
9. They say their good-byes and thank-yous.

CLOSURES

GOOD-BYES AND GIFTS 8

Focus Saying good-bye

Time 10 minutes

Equipment None

Activity

1. Brainstorm toasts from around the world.
2. Mime drinking and saying some of these.
3. Create a special toast for this group.
4. Mime drinking and saying the group toast. Repeat a few times.
5. Say good-byes.

SECTION 3

INFORMATION

USEFUL ADDRESSES

Arts therapies

Arts Therapies Research
c/o Music Therapy
City University
Northampton Square
London EC1V 0HB

Association for Professional Music Therapists
Chestnut Cottage
38 Pierce Lane
Fulbourn
Cambridge
CB1 5DL

British Association for Dramatherapists
5 Sunnydale Villas
Durlston Road
Swanage
Dorset BH19 2HY

British Association of Arts Therapists
11a Richmond Road
Brighton 2BN 3RC

The Association for Dance Movement Therapy
c/o Arts Therapy Department
Springfield Hospital
Glenbourne Road
London SW17 7DJ

Services for older people

Age Concern
277 London Rd
Mitcham
Surrey CR4 3NT
Tel 0181 648 5792

Age Endeavour Fellowship
Willowthorpe
High Street
Stanstead Abbots
Ware
Herts SG12 8AS
Tel 01920 870158

Age Exchange Theatre Trust
11 Blackheath Village
London SE3 9LA
Tel 0181 318 3504

Age Link, Development Officer
29 Penbury Road
Norwood Garden
Southall
Middlesex UB2 5RX
Tel 0181 571 5883

Aged in Distress
54 London Road
Morden
Surrey SM4 5BE
Tel 0181 640 5523

Aged Poor Society
St Joseph's House
42 Brook Green
London W6 7BW

All Party Group of Pensioners
House of Commons
London SW1A DAA
Tel 0171 219 4082

Alzheimer's Disease Society
Gordon House
10 Greencoat Place
London SW1P 1PH
Tel 0171 306 0606

Bedside Manners Theatre Group
Newton Community Care
25 Bertram Street
London N19 5DQ
Tel 0171 281 2526

British Association for Service to the Elderly
119 Hassell Street
Newcastle-under-Lyme
Staffs ST5 1AX
Tel 01782 661033

Contact
15 Henrietta Street
London WC2E HQH
Tel 0171 240 0630

Entertainment Artists' Benevolent Fund
72 Staines Road
Twickenham TW2 5AC
Tel 0181 898 8164

Friends of the Elderly
42 Ebury Street
London SW1 0L2
Tel 0171 730 8263

Help the Aged
St James Walk
London EC1R 0BE
Tel 0171 253 0253

Inter–Acting
33 Gabriel Street
Honor Oak
London SE23 1DW

Jewish Welfare Board
221 Golders Green Road
London NW11 9DW
Tel 0181 458 3282

National Association for Widows
1st Floor, Neville House
14 Waterloo Street
Birmingham B2 5TX

National Trust for the Welfare of the Elderly
33 Hook Road
Goole
Humberside DN14 5JB
Tel 01405 3149

Saga Holidays
The Saga Building
Middleburgh Square
Folkestone
Kent CT20 1AZ
Freephone 0800 300 500

Society for the Relief of Distressed Widows
Nasmith House
175 Tower Bridge Road
London SE1 2AH
Tel 0171 407 7585

University of the Third Age
National Office
1 Stockwell Green
London SW9 9JF
Tel 0171 737 2541

Puppetry

British Unima
The Limes
Norwich Road
Marsham
Norfolk NR10 5PS

London School of Puppetry
2 Ledgard Road
London N5 1DE

Puppetry North West
North West Arts
12 Marter Street
Manchester M1 6MY

Scottish Mask and Puppet Centre
8-10 Bolcannes Avenue
Glasgow G12 0QF

The Puppet Centre BAC
Lavender Hill
London SW11 5TN

Training

There are curently six post graduate training courses which are recognized by the British Association for Dramatherapists. Further information can be obtained by contacting the following institutions.

College of Art & Design
University of Hertfordshire
10 Manor Road
Hatfield AL10 9TL
Tel 01707 285305
(Also MA, higher degrees, advanced courses, Easter and Summer schools)

Department of Counselling
Arden Centre
Sale Road
Northenden
Manchester M23 0DD
Tel 0161 957 1500
(Also some short courses, spring school)

Department of Drama, Film and Television
The University of Ripon & York St John
Lord Mayor's Walk
York YO3 7EX
Tel 01904 656771
(Also short courses, summer school)

Institute of Dramatherapy at Roehampton
The Roehampton Institute
Digby Stuart College
Roehampton Lane
London SW15 5PH
Tel 0181 392 3215/3063
(Also MA, advanced courses, short courses)

SESAME
The Central School of Speech & Drama
Embassy Theatre
Elton Avenue
London NW3 3HY
Tel 0171 722 8183/4/5
(Also short courses)

South Devon College of Arts and Technology
Newton Road
Torquay TW2 5BY
Tel 01803 217589

BIBLIOGRAPHY

Dramatherapy

Gersie A, *Storymaking in Bereavement — Dragons Fight in the Meadow,* Jessica Kingsley, London, 1991.

Gersie A, *Earthtales: Storytelling in Times of Change,* Green Print, London, 1992.

Gersie A & King N, *Storymaking in Education and Therapy,* Jessica Kingsley, London, 1990.

Grainger R, *Drama and Healing: the Roots of Dramatherapy,* Jessica Kingsley, London, 1990.

Jennings S, *Creative Drama in Groupwork,* Winslow Press, Bicester, 1986.

Jennings S (ed.), *Dramatherapy Theory and Practice for Teachers and Clinicians,* Croom Helm, London, 1987.

Jennings S, *Dramatherapy with Families, Groups and Individuals Waiting in the Wings,* Jessica Kingsley, London, 1990.

Jennings S (ed.), *Dramatherapy Theory and Practice II,* Routledge, London, 1992.

Jennings S Cattanach A, Mitchell S, Chesner A & Meldrum B, *Handbook of Dramatherapy,* Routledge, London, 1993.

Landy R, *Persona and Performance: The Meaning of Role in Dramatherapy and Everyday Life,* Jessica Kingsley, London, 1994.

Books of related interest

Boal A, *Games for Actors/Non-actors,* Routledge, London, 1992.

Brun B, Pedersen E & Runbers M, *Symbols of the Soul — therapy and guidance through fairy tales,* Jessica Kingsley, London, 1993.

Bunt L, *Music Therapy — an Art Beyond Words,* Routledge, London, 1994.

Campbell J, *Creative Art in Groupwork,* Winslow Press, Bicester, 1994.

Dynes R, *Creative Games in Groupwork,* Winslow Press, Bicester, 1990.

Dynes R, *Creative Writing in Groupwork,* Winslow Press, Bicester, 1988.

Jennings S & Minde A, *Art Therapy and Dramatherapy — Masks of the Soul,* Jessica Kingsley, London, 1994.

Knights B, *The Listening Reader — fiction and poetry for counsellors and psychotherapists,* Jessica Kingsley, London, 1995.

Liebmann M, *Art Therapy for Groups — a handbook of themes, games and exercises,* Jessica Kingsley, London, 1986.

Meal M (ed.), *Music Therapy in Health and Education,* Jessica Kingsley, London, 1993.

Payne M, *Creative Movement & Dance in Groupwork,* Winslow Press, Bicester, 1990.

Payne M (ed.), *Dance Movement Therapy — Theory and Practice,* Routledge, London, 1992.

Schweitzer P, 'Many happy retirements: an interactive theatre project with older people', Schultzmann P & Clomen-Cruz J (eds), *Playing Boal,* Routledge, London, 1994.

Stuart-Hamilton S, *The Psychology of Ageing — an Introduction,* 2nd edn, Jessica Kingsley, London, 1994.

Therapy and therapeutic activities with elderly people

Bender M, Norris A & Bauckham P, *Groupwork with the Elderly,* Winslow Press, Bicester, 1987.

Bright R, *Music Therapy & the Dementias,* MMB Music Inc, St Louis, Missouri, 1988.

Burnside I, *Working with the Elderly: Group Process and Techniques,* Wordsworth, California, 1994.

Casson J, 'Flying towards Neverland', *Journal of the British Association for Dramatherapists* 16 (2 and 3), 1994.

Cornish P, *Activities for the Frail Aged,* Winslow Press, Bicester, 1987 (out of print).

Daly S, 'Dramatherapy with Elderly People', *Journal of the British Association for Dramatherapists* 11 (2), 1988.

Gersie A, 'Have Your Dream Come True: Mythmaking in therapeutic practice', *Journal of the British Association for Dramatherapists* 7 (2), 1984.

Hanley I & Gilhooly M (eds), *Psychological Therapies for the Elderly,* Croom Helm, London, 1986.

Hanley I & Hodges J (eds), *Psychological Approaches to the Care of the Elderly,* Croom Helm, London, 1984.

Knight B, *Older Adults in Psychotherapy,* Sage, London, 1992.

Murphy G, Langley J *et al*, *Working with Older People: ten training workshops,* Pavilion Publishing, Hove, date unknown.

Neidhart ER & Allen J, *Family Therapy with the Elderly,* Sage, London, 1992.

Stevens S, Le May M, Gravell R & Cook K, *Working with Elderly People: Communication Workshop,* Whurr, London, 1994.

Stokes G & Goudie F (eds), *Working with Dementia,* Winslow Press, Bicester, 1990.

Twining C, *The Memory Handbook,* Winslow Press, Bicester, 1991.

Supervision

Butterworth MC & Faugler J, *Clinical Supervision and Mentorship in Nursing,* Chapman and Hall, London, 1992.

Dryden W and Thorne B, *Training and Supervision for Counselling in Action,* Sage, London, 1991.

Egan G, *The Skilled Helper,* Brooks/Cole Publishing Company, Pacific Grove, California, 1986.

Houston G, *Supervision and Counselling,* Gail Houston, Rochester Foundation, 8 Rochester Terrace, London NW1 9JN, 1990.

Mart GM, *The Process of Clinical Supervision,* University Park Press, Baltimore, 1982.

Pritchard J (ed.), *Good Practice in Supervision — Statutory and Voluntary Organisations,* Jessica Kingsley, London, 1994.

Reminiscence, reality orientation and validation therapies

Castle J, *Reminiscence is Fun!,* 2nd edn, Pavilion Publishing, Hove, 1992.

Feil N, *The Feil Method,* Edward Feil Productions, Cleveland, Ohio, 1982.

Feil N, *The Validation Breakthrough,* Health Professions Press Inc, Baltimore, Maryland, 1993.

Holden U & Woods RT, *Reality Orientation,* Churchill Livingstone, Edinburgh, 1982.

Langley D, *Reminiscence in Dramatherapy and Psychiatry,* Croom Helm, London, 1983.

Langley G & Kershaw B, *'Reminiscence Theatre',* Theatre Paper No 6, Dartington College, Devon, 1982.

Markey M, *Orientation,* Winslow Press, Bicester, 1991.

Norris A, *Reminiscence with Elderly People,* Winslow Press, Bicester, 1986.

Osborn C, *The Reminiscence Handbook,* Age Exchange Publications, London, date unknown.

Rimmer L, *Reality Orientation,* Winslow Press, Bicester, 1982.

Sherman M, *The Reminiscence Quiz Book,* Winslow Press, Bicester, 1991.

Further reading

Arber S (ed.), *Ageing, Independence and the Life Course,* Jessica Kingsley, London, 1993.

Cole T & Winkler M (eds), *Oxford Book of Ageing — Reflections on the Journey of Life,* Oxford University Press, 1984.

De Beauvoir S, *Old Age,* Penguin Books, Harmondsworth, 1977.

Eastwood M (ed.), *Old Age Abuse — A New Perspective,* Chapman and Hall/Age Concern, London, 1994.

Fennel G, Phillipson C & Evers H, *The Society of Old Age,* Open University Press, Milton Keynes, 1988.

Gore I, *Age and Vitality,* Allen & Unwin, London, 1979.

Grainger R, *Change to Life — The pastoral care of the newly retired,* Darton, Longman & Todd, London, 1993.

Johnson J & Slater R (eds), *Ageing and Later Life,* Sage, London, 1983.

Kastenbaum R, *Growing Old,* Harper & Row, London, 1980.

Kroll V, *Growing Older,* Collins, London, 1988.

Pellins M & Smith R, *Life, Death and the Elderly: Historical perspectives,* Routledge, London, 1991.

Walker B, *The Crone, Woman of Age, Wisdom & Power,* Harper & Row, New York, 1985.

Fiction

Balzac H de, trans. Krailseimer A, *Pere Goriot,* Oxford University Press, Oxford, 1991.

Barker P, *The Century's Daughter,* Virago, London, 1986.

Blythe R, *The View in Winter,* Allen Lane, London, 1979.

Comfort A, *A Good Age,* Mitchell Beazley, London, 1977.

Figes E, *Days,* Bloodaxe Books, Newcastle upon Tyne, 1974.

Murdoch I, *The Sandcastle,* Chatto and Windus, London, 1979.

Priestley J, *Instead of the Trees,* Heinemann, London, 1977.

Priestley O, *Over the Long, High Wall,* Heinemann, London, 1972.

Sinclair M, *The Life & Death of Harriet Frean,* Virago, London, 1980.

Spark M, *Memento Mori,* Macmillan, London, 1980.

Tremain R, *Letter to Sister Benedicta,* Hodder & Stoughton, London, 1990.

Tremain R, *Sadler's Birthday,* Hodder & Stoughton, London, 1990.

Plays

Aubrey J, *Brief Lives* (Autobiography & Play), Bookmaster, 1993.

Beckett S, *Endgame,* Faber & Faber, London, 1958.

Beckett S, 'Krapp's Last Tape', 'Rockaby', 'Footfalls', *Collected Shorter Plays of Samuel Beckett,* Faber & Faber, London, 1984.

Chekhov A, 'Uncle Vanya', *Chekhov Plays,* Penguin, Hamondsworth, 1951.

Hilton J, *Goodbye, Mr Chips,* Sceptre, Sevenoaks, 1995.

Mortimer J, *Voyage Round My Father* (Book & Play) French, London, 1972.

Shakespeare W, *King Lear,* various publishers.

ALPHABETICAL LIST OF ACTIVITIES